A CHILD IS BORN

D1545520

A CHILD IS BORN

A natural guide to pregnancy, birth and early childhood

Wilhelm zur Linden, MD

Sophia Books

The information in this book is not intended to be taken as a replacement for medical advice. Persons with a condition requiring medical attention should consult a qualified medical practitioner or suitable therapist.

Sophia Books
Hillside House, The Square
Forest Row, RH18 5ES

www.rudolfsteinerpress.com

Published by Sophia Books 2004
An imprint of Rudolf Steiner Press

First published in English by Rudolf Steiner Press in 1973 with a second edition in 1980. Translated from German by J. Collis. This edition has been edited, updated and revised by Matthew Barton. Originally published in German under the title *Dein Kind* by Vittorio Klostermann, Frankfurt am Main 1975 (12th edition 1986). This English edition includes additions from the comprehensive edition *Geburt und Kindheit*, 1971 (14th edition 1998)

© Vittorio Klostermann GmbH Frankfurt am Main 1971
This translation © Rudolf Steiner Press 2004

A catalogue record for this book is available from the British Library

ISBN 1 85584 192 4

Cover by Andrew Morgan Design
Typeset by DP Photosetting, Aylesbury, Bucks.
Printed and bound in Great Britain by Cromwell Press Ltd., Trowbridge, Wilts.

Contents

PUBLISHER'S NOTE

Most of the preparations, medicines and products mentioned in this book are available throughout the English-speaking world. In case of difficulty, some useful website addresses are listed below:

Weleda: www.weleda.com *or* www.weleda.co.uk
Wala: www.wala.de
Holle baby foods: www.holle.de

The author's recommendation of medicines and other products arises out of his personal experience as a paediatrician and general practitioner, and in no way constitutes an advertisement.

Measurements:
British 'dessertspoon' = American 'soupspoon' or 'table-spoon'.
British 'tablespoon' = American 'serving spoon'.
(The British terms are used in this book.)

Foreword

When Wilhelm zur Linden died on 5 December 1972, the ninth edition of this book was in preparation. He always stressed the importance of keeping abreast of contemporary issues and current needs, and was continually at pains to update his research. This had been an important factor for him when he first conceived the book, determining its character and content from the beginning. This striving to keep his finger on the pulse was enhanced by his astute approach to themes and problems. Drawing on rich life experience, with compassion and wisdom, he succeeded in formulating things in a way that is still valid and innovative today. Much that zur Linden stated in his own day, which met with great resistance, has meanwhile become a matter of course—such as his recommendations for gentler birth techniques, his reservation about vaccinations and his opposition to Vigantol (synthetic vitamin D) treatment.

Although the scientific world view underpinning modern medicine has produced results of major importance in combating illness, it is simply not adequate on its own for an unprejudiced understanding of all the processes and transformations that occur at conception, and during pregnancy, birth and the child's further development. One has to acknowledge, in fact, that science itself often does not fully understand the knowledge it has acquired through the microscope and the dissecting knife, and that its limited, more mechanistic perspectives give rise to a lack of clear direction, for instance in relation to birth control, gene technology, extending life expectancy etc. The human body cannot be understood in terms of itself alone, but only acquires sense as an instrument of the spirit which inhabits it. It will hopefully become apparent to the reader that the approach represented in this book, in contrast to the purely scientific outlook, not only makes sense but is also extraordinarily practical and beneficial.

The living and developing nature of this book, expressed not least in increasing demand for it, has faced the publisher with the task of extending it as Wilhelm zur Linden would have wished, supervising new editions and integrating new knowledge and findings. The book is today used even more extensively than in the past, since generally valid guidelines on questions surrounding birth, care of the child, nutrition and education are no longer passed on from one generation to the next as a matter of course, but each person now has to find his or her own answers. It is true that in the meantime a certain awareness has developed of environmental and nutritional issues, but at the same time greater threats have arisen, some of which—such as television and ubiquitous computer technology—have not yet generally been recognized as such. To really understand human childhood and to apply different standards to this phase of life than we do to adulthood has become one of the most important contemporary issues. This book aims to spur readers to become aware of these issues which we encounter on a daily basis. It offers help in dealing with them, inviting us to use our capacity for empathy, our imagination and our healthy common sense. It is therefore not just a handbook offering ready-made solutions but a guide that urges us to think and act. It is intended less for a single reading than for ongoing reference, in other words for repeated and living engagement with its content.

Günther Schönemann, MD
Brigitte Schönemann, née zur Linden

Introduction

The uniqueness of every child

We know that the protein substance of which almost the whole body is composed is structured differently in each one of us. Likewise we know that the skin profile image which we are familiar with as fingerprint is wholly unique in each individual on this earth; and that even the fine structure of our hair is distinct from that of all other people.

In contrast to the plant world, where young plants do not deviate at all from others of the same species, and in contrast to animals whose young show no marked differences in form from their parents, we find in the infant, and even in many newborn babies, bodily forms such as the ear, or even unique inner characteristics, that do not appear in the same way anywhere else in the family or in previous generations. Even in families with many children there are the greatest differences between siblings, and this means that we must nowadays bring up our children in very individual ways. We cannot even feed them according to general recommendations without ignoring their uniqueness. From birth already, babies react in very distinct and individual ways.

It is therefore more important to find out what is new and unique in our children's nature—and when this new element is valuable to help it develop fully—than, as is common today, to consider inherited characteristics as of prime importance. Not in what is already known and handed down within the family, but in the new element that every child brings into the world does the unique possibility lie for new energies, capacities or ideas to be realized, which our world so urgently needs. Each child born might develop into an individual who helps humanity forwards in decisive ways, showing it new paths towards a light-filled ascent from contemporary confusion. Innovative geniuses have often sprung from fairly unremarkable families!

By focusing on the uniqueness of every child, in fact of every human being, we come to the following discovery: in the plant world, given the same conditions, the offspring plant is as like the mother plant as 'two peas in a pod'. In the animal world each member of a species resembles the others as far as physical and soul characteristics are concerned. In the most highly developed mammals there are certain differences between members of a species, but these are not fundamental in nature.

When we come to the human being we find, despite certain similarities between people, that there is no point in speaking of genus or type, for each individual is in some sense a species in himself. He has life processes and metabolic forces in common with his fellow human beings; he has soul impulses similar to those that move the souls of others. But above and beyond this he also possesses the spark of spirit, whose nature and striving is different in each individual, making every person distinct and unique.

It is this spark of spirit which makes the soul think, feel and have impulses of will in a very particular way. Even the metabolic processes are different in each person as a result. The spirit also expresses itself in the gestures of our hands and our gait, and determines the unique structure of every cell in our body.

When we attempt to explain the wholly new and unique element that each child bears within him,★ we touch on one of the greatest mysteries of human life.

Unusual events mostly happen at special places and under very special conditions. This is also true of the interior of the womb. Without any exaggeration one can say that conditions reign in the womb which one only otherwise finds on or even above the highest mountain peaks of the earth, in the cosmos. The developing embryo must live and develop with a very small supply of oxygen. His red blood count and blood colour, the whole composition of his blood, corresponds to these conditions. We adults would immediately lose consciousness and die if we lived like this.

The body of the developing embryo is embedded in the mother's body in a wonderful way, receiving ideal protection. Apart from the wall of the placenta, the embryo is also enveloped in the so-called foetal membranes. These membranes are extremely important for the developing child because as the embryo grows they play a part in the gradual uniting of the child's soul and spirit with the body. At birth their task is complete and they are then discarded as 'after-birth'. The work of the placenta is similar. This is an organ filled with the mother's blood, which serves to nourish the child. At the same time it acts as a filter, so that the stream of nourishment does not flow directly from the mother's organism to the embryo.

★ To avoid the awkwardness of using both genders, we will alternate from chapter to chapter (Ed.).

Thus the embryo is carried, protected and nourished by the mother, and yet its development and growth takes place for the most part quite separately from the mother's organism. The membranes and placenta in many ways isolate it from the life of the mother. Floating in the waters of the womb, the embryo is barely subject to gravity. Furthermore it contains an extremely small proportion of firm mineral substance: at 3 to 4 months the embryo consists of 93 per cent water and even at birth it is still 80 per cent fluid, thus only a fifth of it consists of solid matter.

If one tries to understand these facts then one comes to see that the developing child in the womb needs quite different conditions before birth than it does afterwards. Before birth the child is not yet really an earthly being, but one embedded in the cosmos and its forces.

Describing the mystery of birth in olden times, myths spoke of the stork who brings babies. The fairy tales of all cultures speak of the help given to mankind by white birds such as swans, doves and storks. These white birds are a pictorial description of beings who create a link between the spiritual and earthly world. So in the stork we have a picture of the human ego being carried from heaven to earth. For our forefathers this was obviously the decisive process, more important than the physical and physiological aspects of birth.

This picture of the child coming down to us is the basis for the wonder and reverence with which we can approach the new 'arrival'. Parents, after all, are no more than helpers in this marvellous event in which a spiritual being unites with an earthly body formed by an act of divine creation and placed at that spirit's service for a whole lifetime.

1

The Growing Embryo

Expecting the child

Conception is often a deep, inner experience, something that may even be sensed before a woman consciously knows she is pregnant—perhaps in the form of a powerful and joyful dream.

Fortunately most women when they discover they are pregnant are far more delighted with the prospect than alarmed at the mysterious process now going on within their body. But even so, lack of knowledge or faulty information often lead to anxiety and may be the source of some of the problems of pregnancy. This book is intended to provide the answers to many questions about pregnancy, birth and diet, and care of the infant and small child.

Signs of pregnancy

Women who menstruate regularly can be fairly sure they are pregnant if a monthly period fails to occur; and if the following period also fails to appear, a pregnancy is virtually certain. With healthy women whose menstruation is irregular, the missing of one or several periods is not a sure sign of pregnancy. They should consult their doctor about possible blood or urine tests which can give early certainty, or purchase a test kit at the chemist. The doctor can also determine a pregnancy of six weeks or more by internal examination, which is preferable to an ultrasound scan. Some believe the latter to have potentially adverse effects on the developing embryo.

Further signs, in addition to the cessation of menstruation, are enlargement of the breasts, their secretion of small amounts of colostrum (a yellowish fluid which precedes the formation of milk after the baby is born), morning nausea or sickness, frequent urge to pass water, and excessive weariness in the evening. Some women, however, feel particularly healthy and vigorous when pregnant and do not suffer from tiredness or nausea.

The final and unmistakable signs of pregnancy do not occur till the fifth month, when the mother feels the baby's movements for the first time and when the doctor can hear the baby's heartbeat with his stethoscope and feel the different parts of the embryo.

Expected date of birth

To calculate the probable date of the baby's birth, women with a normal menstrual cycle of 28 days should take the first day of their last period, subtract three months and add seven days. This will give the date in the following year when the baby may be expected. For example: Last regular period started 5 November; three months earlier 5 August; add seven days and the probable date of birth will be 12 August in the following year.

However, this rule of thumb must be taken as a very rough guide only, since every child has his own, for him normal, needs which determine the length of pregnancy. The average is 280 to 282 days or ten lunar months, though one usually speaks of nine calendar months or forty weeks.

The baby's movements can first be felt almost exactly in the middle of a first pregnancy. In a second or subsequent pregnancy the movements are felt 12 to 14 days earlier.

Medical examination during pregnancy

The expectant mother should see her gynaecologist for an examination after the sixth week of pregnancy. He will want to check her blood pressure, blood count (possible anaemia) and kidney activity, and also ascertain that her pelvis will allow the baby to pass through the birth canal. (For instance, a malformed pelvis, possibly due to rickets, could present an obstacle.)

Even if the first examination is satisfactory, the mother should see the gynaecologist regularly throughout the pregnancy. She should inform him about illnesses in the family such as epilepsy or diabetes and also about any acute feverish illnesses she may have had. He must be notified of any bleeding from the vagina immediately, even if it seems insignificant. Regarding the *rhesus factor* see pages 14–15 and regarding *vaccination* during pregnancy see pages 10–11 and 157.

Alongside these physical examinations, the mother's emotional state should not be forgotten. By patiently answering the questions that may now assail her, the doctor can help her achieve the emotional calm and stability that is so beneficial to the developing embryo.

Ailments of pregnancy

Pregnancy can be the cause of trivial and sometimes also more serious ailments, especially if the expectant mother is in some way unable to adjust to her new situation or cope with the greater demands made on her. Quite independently from this, however, a mother may be plagued by discomforts in her first pregnancy and free of them during the second, and vice versa.

Morning nausea or sickness, when only gastric juices and hardly ever food are brought up, does not lead to loss of weight. Relief can often be achieved by chewing some raw oat flakes. It is also helpful to drink two to three cups of Weleda Pinella tea daily (or any other herbal tea specified for liver and gall). Sometimes, however, there is serious and prolonged vomiting of the food eaten. In these cases the doctor should be consulted, since there is usually also lack of appetite, and considerable weight loss can ensue. Great care must be taken to correct resulting deficiencies in mineral salts (iron, calcium) and vitamins.

For *heartburn* it is helpful to take Weleda Digestodoron (20 drops 3 times daily). Alternatively one can chew a few hazel or cashew nuts till they become a tasteless pulp in the mouth. When this is swallowed it controls the gastric acids.

Excessive flow of saliva plagues some expectant mothers: sometimes more than a litre (two pints) a day is produced. This can often be improved by chewing very well on a few dried juniper berries.

Swellings on face or legs should definitely be shown to the doctor (take a sample of early morning urine). If he finds the cause to be merely congestion, Weleda Skin Tone Lotion rubbed into the skin is a good remedy.

Excessive tiredness can frequently be caused by anaemia, and should therefore be investigated. It is wrong, however, to take any iron preparation without first undergoing a blood test. The same applies to other medicines, vitamin preparations, etc. Synthetic vitamin D in any form should be avoided. If anaemia is diagnosed, it should be treated immediately. This is also important in the case of any circulatory weakness.

Difficulty in breathing, particularly during the last three months, can be caused by the increasing lack of space in the abdomen. It is a help to breathe calmly and deeply in and out (particularly out!).

Palpitations (which sometimes accompany breathlessness) and *pains in the sciatic nerve* do not usually require any special treatment.

Congestion of blood in the veins of the legs, which causes *varicose veins*, should be treated. Apart from taking certain medicines for the circulation, it is often a help to bandage the legs with elastic bandages or to wear support stockings.

Constipation must definitely be avoided. The following is a useful recipe: In the evening, soak in half a pint (quarter of a litre) of cold water one dessertspoon each of wheat bran, wheat germ and whole linseed together with one or two chopped figs or prunes. Eat this either cold or heated for breakfast the next morning.

Depressive moods and even thoughts of suicide, also rapid changes of mood, belong to the difficulties experienced by some women in pregnancy. They are rarely serious and usually pass without treatment. The same goes for unusual *cravings* for certain foods and acute *dislike* of others.

Piles and *varicose vulva* are difficulties experienced frequently in pregnancy and can cause the expectant mother great discomfort, quite overshadowing the happy mood which should prevail during her time of waiting. Women who remain at work well into pregnancy are particularly prone to these afflictions, which are caused by circulatory congestion in the abdomen. The doctor can and must help. In less serious cases Weleda Stibium 0.4% Suppositories for piles are helpful. They contain a remedy which stimulates the circulation. A daily and easy movement of the bowels is also essential (see recipe above). It can also be helpful to sit in a cold bath for six seconds (not longer!) every evening, after which one wraps the lower part of the body in a Turkish towel and goes to bed without drying.

Stretch marks appear on the mother's abdomen, and sometimes even on breasts and thighs, as her girth increases. These can remain visible after the birth of the baby and should be rubbed with a good skin oil.

Patches like freckles can appear on the mother's face, but these disappear on their own after the birth of the baby.

Threats to the embryo

Among the most frequent causes of malformation are abortion attempts, either with instruments or by chemical means.

With some virus infections (especially German measles, but also mumps, chicken pox and Asian flu) there is a danger that the virus might pass from the mother's to the child's blood. If this happens, malformations are especially likely in the first three months. The same applies to smallpox vaccination (see page 157), which should therefore be avoided during pregnancy, especially during the first three and in the final months. Live oral vaccination against polio should be avoided, particularly during the early months. Treatment with BCG vaccine against tuberculosis is only recommended if the expectant mother has unavoidable, close contact with a patient suffering from open tuberculosis where isolation is impossible.

The thalidomide tragedy has shown the dangers of sleeping pills. And of course thalidomide is not the only substance that can cripple the embryo. Doctors all over the world agree that the unchecked use of pills of all kinds constitutes an increasing threat to health, and this threat is magnified in pregnancy.

Large doses of hormones, for instance cortisone, taken during the first three months of pregnancy, have been shown to cause serious malformations such as cleft lip and cleft palate.

An expectant mother must not be allowed to undergo any kind of X-ray examination or treatment on any part of the body except in life-or-death situations. The same applies of course to radiotherapy of all kinds.

There are a number of other diseases and environmental causes that can damage the embryo. Among these are venereal diseases and certain parasites such as canine tapeworms. Shocks should be avoided. An unbalanced and qualitatively inferior diet can have undesirable consequences. Radioactive contamination of food and drinking water is an environmental threat whose consequences for future generations cannot yet be accurately foreseen.

Morning sickness does not on the whole affect the embryo, but babies whose mothers have experienced serious sickness during pregnancy should be carefully examined and kept under observation for several years by their doctor.

Smoking during pregnancy and breastfeeding

Since smoking is still on the increase, the subject cannot be omitted from a book of this kind.

There should certainly be no smoking when babies and small children are in the room. It has been shown that the pulse of an unborn child accelerates after only a few inhalations by the mother, and nursing mothers can even cause nicotine poisoning in their babies, for nicotine is one of the strongest poisons known to us.

Recent research has shown that the amount of vitamin C in the milk of smoking mothers is considerably lower than in that of mothers who do not smoke. It was found in addition that this lack of vitamin C could not be corrected by the consumption of either additional citrus fruit or vitamin C tablets. This is another way in which smoking by expectant and nursing mothers damages the child, for the baby needs a great deal of vitamin C, especially in winter and spring.

Many smokers repeatedly attempt to break this habit. An expectant or nursing mother is responsible not only for herself but also for a growing human being, her child. There is only one effective measure with which to combat addiction to nicotine: give up smoking today.

Alcohol during pregnancy and breastfeeding

The child is always at risk if a mother drinks alcohol while pregnant. This can lead to malformations of the embryo, not only in seriously alcohol-dependent mothers. The incompletely developed liver of the unborn child cannot break down the alcohol that penetrates through the placenta boundary.

All of the child's organs can suffer damage as a result: children can be born small and only grow slowly after birth. Mental and motor development may be delayed, often due to severe changes in the brain. Heart defects can manifest, kidney and genital malformations can arise, and also skeletal deformations. The body of a child is thus damaged in a way that makes it harder for his individual spirit to unite with it. For this reason a pregnant woman should avoid all alcohol both during pregnancy and while breastfeeding, for the alcohol also passes into the child through the milk.

Drugs

Young people and even children are increasingly taking drugs of all kinds. Young pregnant women, therefore, may take drugs or even be addicted. For the 'softer' drugs the same applies as for alcohol, coffee and nicotine—mothers need to be aware of the risks involved and the potential harm to the foetus. Hard drugs are a still graver danger. Many children are already born addicted to drugs such as heroin, and, besides the lasting health problems arising from this, they suffer severe withdrawal symptoms during their first weeks of life. All that is possible should be done to help mothers relinquish drug habits early in pregnancy.

German measles

This childhood illness, which is otherwise associated with little risk, can cause damage to the eyes, ears and heart of the embryo if the mother is infected with it during the first three months of pregnancy. Fortunately malformations occur in only a relatively low number of such cases. However, women who are not sure if they had German measles when they were children should undergo a test to find out and discuss vaccination with their doctor if the result is negative.

Toxoplasmosis

A minute parasite in the mother's blood penetrates the placenta and invades the blood of the embryo, which either dies or, less frequently, suffers severe damage mainly to the nervous system, in which inflammation is generated. Usually severe and irreversible damage is done to the brain, eyes or ears.

The parasites are transferred to the mother from domestic animals, dogs, cats, rabbits, sheep, pigeons and animals bred for their fur. Pregnant women who have contact with these creatures should be examined even if they themselves do not feel ill. Early treatment can prevent damage to the child.

This illness is becoming more frequent and it is advisable to undergo a blood test before contemplating pregnancy.

The rhesus factor

Research using the blood of rhesus monkeys has revealed that many miscarriages are connected with certain characteristics of the red blood corpuscles. The blood of about 85% of the population is 'rhesus positive', while that of the remainder is 'rhesus negative'. If both parents are the same, either positive or negative, or if the mother is rhesus positive and the father rhesus negative, there is nothing to worry about.

But if the father is rhesus positive and the mother rhesus negative it can be a problem if the baby inherits the father's positive factor. In such cases it is possible for some of the baby's rhesus positive blood to enter the mother's blood-stream via the placenta, whereupon her system will start to make antibodies to combat the 'foreign' blood, either during pregnancy or after the birth. Though this does not usually affect the first child, subsequent children can be seriously harmed: the destruction of the red blood corpuscles leads to acute anaemia, or a fatal attack of jaundice immediately after birth, or severe brain damage.

These babies can be saved by a complete exchange of blood within six hours of birth, a method which has so far shown no damaging side effects.

Parents who are in this difficult position can take certain steps to minimize the problem. The mother herself should avoid having blood transfusions if at all possible, but in an emergency the blood she is given must be carefully selected, taking into account not only her blood group but also the rhesus factor. It is feared that even fairly frequent intramuscular injections of blood can sensitize the recipient's blood, so in these cases, too, the rhesus factor must be taken into account. (The whole problem has nothing to do with ordinary blood groups.)

The mother should eat plenty of citrus fruit which has a high vitamin C content and should take care that her calcium count is sufficiently high (but not by taking vitamin D!). These two factors will help reduce the brittleness of the tiny blood vessels, thus helping to prevent any of the child's blood from escaping through the placenta into her bloodstream.

There is now also an anti-rhesus serum which is injected into the mother immediately after the birth as a protection for a future child.

Down's Syndrome

The relative frequency of Down's Syndrome children born to older parents is probably less to do with their greater age than with the fact that such people may have damaged their genetic stock in the course of their lives through various factors such as poor diet, X-rays or even drugs. It is quite wrong to cause anxiety to every older, pregnant woman with such 'knowledge', since there is no hard and fast rule about this. Amniocentesis tests undertaken shortly before birth to ascertain a disorder should only be carried out in urgent cases on the advice of a doctor, due to the considerable risk to the embryo.

Parents who have given birth to a Down's Syndrome child should take heart, trying to perceive the true nature of their special child and their task in relation to him. Such children are often experienced as very loving, sunny people, who bring much joy to their families.

If the family cannot cope, there are many homes and villages for children in need of special care, based on the work of Rudolf Steiner, where they can be nurtured and even learn appropriate skills and professions.

Avoiding miscarriage

During the first three months and from the seventh month of pregnancy, miscarriages or premature births are not too unusual, particularly in the case of a first pregnancy or when there has been a previous miscarriage. During the remaining months, miscarriage is also possible but less likely.

As a normal precaution one should avoid heavy carrying,

lifting or stretching (e.g. hanging up washing) and also squatting for any length of time. Long rides in buses or cars and riding on motor cycles should be avoided because of the shaking and jarring these cause.

The expectant mother should have plenty of rest, going to bed early and lying down for one or two hours after lunch. She should undress and relax completely in bed.

Strong laxatives are to be avoided and constipation treated by adhering to the right diet taken with sufficient water. Laxative teas are also useful, for example Weleda Clairo Tea taken not too strong. See also the recipe mentioned in the section on *Ailments of pregnancy*, page 9.

The danger to the child if the mother smokes during pregnancy is discussed on pages 11–12.

If there is any danger of a miscarriage, marital intercourse should be avoided, particularly when the monthly periods would be due.

Any movement which disturbs the natural rhythms of the organism is unfavourable, for instance typing, sewing by machine and many other machine jobs, if they have to be carried out for hours on end. Occupations which require sitting with the upper part of the body bent forward are also unsuitable.

During pregnancy one should not totally immerse oneself in any activity, even such household chores as stirring, winding wool or knitting. The many-sided activity of the housewife is really the most suited to pregnancy so long as nothing is overdone. But the housewife should not think that her work in the house or even her walks to the shops can be a substitute for regular carefree walks when she tries to let nothing weigh on her mind.

Signs of danger

Pregnant women are safeguarded against many dangers as though they were under a special mantle of protection. On the whole they do not succumb to ordinary illnesses and the majority feel particularly well, better than at any other time in their lives. They are fitter, more balanced and more resistant to infection and illness.

It is therefore more as a precautionary measure and for reassurance that a number of symptoms are listed below about which the doctor should be consulted without delay. (It is a good idea to take a sample of early morning urine with you when you go for a consultation):

- bleeding resembling that of the monthly period even if less profuse. If this occurs one should go straight to bed and lie on one's back, keeping the legs quite still, until the doctor arrives;
- excessive nausea and vomiting after the third month and serious faintness;
- swelling of hands, ankles and eyelids;
- weight increases of more than two pounds (one kilogram) per month.

Sport during pregnancy

The best 'sport' during pregnancy is the mother's regular daily walk, but she should remember that in the later months a quarter of an hour's physical activity is equivalent to an hour when not pregnant. Swimming can also be encouraged during the first half of pregnancy if the water is not too cold or the waves too high. But the expectant mother should not dive or swim under water.

It is best to avoid eurythmy, gymnastics, skiing, tennis, athletics, and anything else which requires strenuous muscular exertion or jarring of the body. If possible the mother should not subject herself to extreme changes of altitude, whether by travelling from low-lying parts into high mountains or vice versa, or by flying.

As the baby grows, the mother will find her breathing becoming increasingly shallow and she might feel short of breath. A simple breathing exercise can be helpful. Stand by an open window wearing a loose dress. Breathe in and out through the nose, taking care particularly to empty the lungs completely on the out-breath. Do not, however, pause before breathing in again, nor before breathing out when the lungs are quite filled. Raise the arms lightly on the in-breath and lower them on the out-breath. Ten long breaths like this three times daily should suffice.

The doctor will advise on special gymnastics suitable for pregnancy. The most important thing is to avoid excesses of any kind.

Diet during pregnancy

Those who normally have a varied diet of good quality food need not change their ways much when pregnant. Within reason one can eat what one pleases and even yield to any cravings one might suddenly have. It is important to have regular meals and better to add an extra meal rather than eat too much at a time.

The expectant mother should be very careful about the amount of tea and coffee she drinks. The same applies to maté tea which contains a considerable amount of caffeine.

The soft drinks now on the market which contain caffeine are also unsuitable. In addition to caffeine they contain a number of undesirable chemicals, the most dubious being orthophosphoric acid, which provides the stimulating effect. This acid can damage the liver, particularly as the advertisements advise that these drinks should be taken ice cold. As we have seen, alcohol and smoking are out of the question during pregnancy. Hot spices should not be used either.

Our diet these days usually contains too much protein, so the expectant mother should take eggs, meat and fish in small quantities only. An egg a day is absolute nonsense, and eggs which are more than eight or ten days old have lost much of their nutritional value anyway. The meat eaten should where possible be that of young animals.

When changing to a vegetarian diet, care must be taken to ensure that deficiencies, especially of protein, do not arise. Normal protein needs can be met with curd cheese (see recipe page 199), cottage cheese, milk and cereals. Vegetables should be as free as possible of chemical additives and other impurities, and vegetables that cause flatulence (such as cabbage and dried pulses) should be avoided.

As a general guide it can be said that during the first three months Bircher muesli and sour fruits are excellent foods, whereas too many pastry and farinaceous dishes should be avoided.

During the second three-month period sweet fruits, particularly from southern countries (including almonds), are particularly beneficial.

And during the last three months all kinds of cereals are good because of their mineral content (wheat, barley, green rye, millet and, to a lesser extent, oats).

The daily food of an expectant mother should include: high-quality dark rye bread, at least half a pint (quarter of a litre) of milk daily in any form (including yogurt, sour milk, buttermilk, kefir), fresh vegetables, every kind of salad (e.g. lettuce, lamb's lettuce, endive, cress, cucumber), fruit in season, and fresh herbs daily if possible (parsley, chives, sweet basil, savory, fennel, lovage, thyme, marjoram) or powdered if not available fresh. They can be grown in the kitchen in flower pots if necessary.

Recent research (G.A. Winter and others) suggests that it is the substances and forces found in herbs such as these which gave our parents and grandparents their greater resistance to infections of various kinds, so our modern susceptibility to infections of all sorts is reason enough to pay more attention once again to these herbs.

It is often believed in error that plenty of fruit can be a substitute for vegetables. But vegetables contain indispensable mineral salts which are not found in fruit.

Regular bowel habits go hand in hand with the right dietary habits. The right kind of bread is a particular help here and many suitable breads can be obtained in delicatessen and health food shops, for instance lactose bread, waerland bread, Demeter bread, Steinmetz bread, pumpernickel, dark breads baked in wood ovens. Bread should not be eaten too fresh. Organic, wholegrain wheat flakes, obtainable in health food shops, are also good.

Constipation can also arise as a result of too little fluid being taken. Herb teas, fruit juices and elixirs (Sandthorn, Rose Hip, Blackthorn, etc.) should be taken instead of milk, which can often cause constipation and flatulence.

Care of teeth for mother and child

It is often said that every child costs the mother a tooth. This is quite untrue if the right precautions are taken, even though the child does need a great deal of calcium and other salts. It is, however, a mistake to imagine that calcium or vitamin tablets can help. In the milk, cheese, bread, vegetables and even often the drinking water of a healthy diet there is more calcium than is required daily by the human organism. It is the ability to absorb the calcium which is disturbed in many people and which leads to a calcium deficiency in the blood. Then the calcium taken in tablet form is excreted along with the calcium in the daily food. Thus the greater need for calcium that arises through pregnancy remains unsatisfied. The expectant mother's saliva lacks the ability to protect the teeth from the acids arising in her mouth from bacterial activity in remnants of food.

Calcium taken in homoeopathic doses gradually stimulates the impaired ability to absorb calcium, so that the organism can learn once again to take in the necessary amounts for mother and baby from the food eaten. Many doctors find Weleda Calcium Supplements I and II particularly effective.

Essential for proper care of the teeth is a small toothbrush that can reach even the awkward crevices. Nylon bristles are preferred, as natural bristle collects bacteria too easily. The toothpaste used should not contain chemical disinfectants. Recommended are Weleda dental creams and saline paste.

Preparing physically for the birth of the baby

Pregnancy is not an illness, indeed often it is a time of enhanced physical well-being. Those who already live sensibly and healthily need not make many changes in their way of life.

Care of the skin is important during pregnancy. Weleda skin lotions are stimulating and refreshing and can be used daily. Brushing with a dry brush or loofah also stimulates the circulation in the right way.

Women should not take warm baths more than twice a week and during pregnancy these should not be warmer than 97°F (36°C). Weleda pine and lavender bath milks may be added.

During the ninth month one can prepare for the birth by taking a hipbath with lime blossom tea every other day: pour two pints (1 litre) of boiling water on a handful of lime blossoms, cover and allow to infuse for five minutes and then strain. Add this to the hipbath, which should not be hotter than 99°F (37°C). Stay in the bath for about ten minutes at first, but during the last two weeks for five minutes only.

Sunbathing should be undertaken with extreme caution and never for long periods at a time. Use a good herbal lotion for protecting the skin.

Early care of the nipples is important. If they are rather flat they should be drawn out gently night and morning. A milk pump can be used for this if they are too flat. Unsuitable non-porous brassieres often damage the nipples and cause them to lose their natural firmness. During the later months of pregnancy they should be rubbed daily with a few drops of lemon juice to help them regain their proper firmness. Oil or a greasy cream should only be used occasionally, otherwise the surface becomes too flabby.

The breasts themselves also lose their firmness when brassieres are too tight. A brief daily massage, rubbing from the base to the nipple, will help strengthen them and they should now be allowed to develop freely so that they will not lose shape through breastfeeding.

The importance of regular bowel habits in preparation for the baby's birth has already been discussed. This can be achieved with the right diet (see pages 19–21).

Expectant mothers usually have a great need for sleep and should have ten hours a night and at least one hour in the middle of the day, when they should undress and go to bed properly.

Daily walks in the fresh air have already been mentioned.

Marital intercourse can do no harm until about eight weeks before the birth is expected, but should be strictly avoided if there is any danger of miscarriage.

It is unwise during pregnancy to subject oneself to any great changes in altitude, for instance holidays in the mountains if one lives in a lowland area. Flying is also best avoided.

When sitting, the legs should not be crossed, as this considerably impairs the circulation.

Psychological preparation for the baby's arrival

It is essential during the whole of pregnancy to practise what might be called soul hygiene. The baby cannot flourish if the mother's soul is filled with worry and anxiety, but he thrives if she is filled with calm happiness and anticipation. A depressed mood causes cramped breathing, which in turn leads to many organic disturbances.

Particularly important is the avoidance of shocks of any kind. Cinema and television are thus unsuitable entertainment during pregnancy, since any moment something might be shown which could cause an unexpected shock.

Pregnancy is not a time for seeking diversions but rather a period of life which calls for an inner concentration of all one's soul forces on the happy event which is soon to take place. As a help in this inner collecting of thoughts and feelings, Rudolf Steiner often suggested that expectant mothers might contemplate a beautiful picture. He particularly recommended the Madonna pictures by Raphael, above all the Sistine Madonna. Contemplating this in peace and feeling its content in her soul, the mother will soon discover the helpful strength such a picture can give.

While the expectant mother need not burden her soul with all sorts of weighty problems, pondering seriously on the fundamental questions of life and also her responsibility towards the child she is expecting can enhance her basic mood of joyous expectation.

Preparing older siblings for the arrival

It is important to speak to the other children in the family about the expected baby as early as possible and they may like to feel the baby moving inside 'mummy's tummy'. There is nothing wrong in telling them the old tale of the stork who brings down the child's soul from heaven. This will not contradict for them the fact of the baby growing inside their mother's body, for children have a natural understanding of the truths which the wisdom of ancient times clothed in pictures such as that of the stork.

If told about the expected baby in the right way, the older children are sure to share in this happy expectation and they will do their best to be good when they know that their mother is carrying the child. It is indeed their right to share in the preparations, for after all, the new arrival will be their own brother or sister, theirs to protect and look after.

In the case of a home confinement it is best to send the older children away for a few days if possible, but as soon as they return they should not be neglected, otherwise they may become jealous. They should be allowed to participate in and watch everything, particularly feeding. This brings a harmonious atmosphere into the life of the family, especially if they are also allowed to perform small tasks for the new baby.

Family experiences like these help in forming character and they provide the foundation for the development of a responsible attitude towards other human beings later on.

2

Problems of Contraception

The problem of birth control or contraception is many-layered and not solely a medical issue.

Naturally the exponential increase in the world population, and overpopulation in some areas can be regarded as a threat to mankind. In Europe, too, we cannot avoid the issue of ethically acceptable means of birth control. Since the discovery of chemical or hormonal birth control methods, however, the problem seems to have become an arbitrary process. These new possibilities of preventing conception actually mean that we should be more not less conscious in preparing to become parents. Then they can extend our scope for freedom of action and enhance our moral responsibility.

For many parents the method of refraining from intercourse on fertile days is recommended, with the proviso, however, that it is of only limited use for women with irregular or very short cycles. If the time extending from the first day of menses to the first day of the next menses is only about 21 days, and menstruation itself lasts 5 or 6 days, the end of menstruation falls in the fertile time. Ovulation occurs 15 days before the next menstruation, 21 minus 15 gives 6: in other words the infertile time extends only from the 10th to the 21st day. It is therefore wrong to think that the first days after menstruation are always infertile. In such cases it is advisable to measure basal temperature. In doing so one must always remember that while the egg can only be fertilized over about six hours, the sperm cell remains capable of fertilization for roughly three days. This means that a slightly shifted ovulation time can easily lead to conception. It is best for couples to consult a gynaecologist about this, who will be able to advise on the best method of contraception.

Contraception using hormones, that is, the contraceptive pill, is a method which, in my view, the doctor can only prescribe with great caution. Previous experience has shown that it disrupts hormonal balance and thus, linked to this, our emotional life. There may be robust women who do not suffer much in consequence. In more sensitive ones, in contrast, the resulting complaints are often so considerable that they soon stop taking the pill. Symptoms can include insomnia, nervous irritability, or coldness towards their partner and aversion to sexual intercourse. Sometimes women suffer aching veins and thyroid complaints. There may also be cravings for all foods, particularly sweet ones, and an undesired increase in weight. In general women feel they have changed in their intrinsic nature, which is also the case where other hormones are taken. Cases have been described where the husband became impotent when his wife took the pill. Married life is often disrupted and disturbed.

The increased tendency to embolism is particularly a problem. Severe brain infarcts with peripheral paralysis can occur, particularly after delivery.

Pharmacologists also fear damage to any future children. Younger women should definitely not take the pill for more than a short period.

One frequently hears reports of multiple births that occur after women stop taking the pill. All this seems to suggest that the pill is a 'crime against nature'. Many young couples thankfully decide not to take the contraceptive pill until they have had their third child.

The gynaecologist must decide whether a pessary is a good idea. This closes the cervix and must be changed every month, which often dictates against its use.

There are a wide variety of chemical contraceptives available, such as sprays and creams for application to the vagina, which aim to kill the sperm. In general one can say that these chemical contraceptives are uncertain and also risk damaging a child who is, nevertheless, conceived. The growing number of children damaged at the embryo stage should be a warning against imperfectly effective and health-damaging preventive methods.

The doctor should also warn against the *coitus interruptus* method. This gives rise to dissatisfaction on both sides, which can ultimately lead to an aversion towards each other, and can trigger nervous disorders in both men and women.

Surgical methods, involving tying off the fallopian tube in women or the sperm tubes in the man, usually leads to complete sterilization.

Implantation of a so-called *coil* in the womb is also problematic. It is true that this does not result in lasting sterility, but may have health repercussions and is morally debatable since its effect is similar to continual, mechanical abortion at an early stage.

In many cases the doctor must therefore resort to advising use of a condom, although it is best if a couple's whole situation can be considered first, to see if this is really the most appropriate means of contraception. There are some reports of emotional problems linked to condom use. Outside of

marriage, particularly, condoms have great hygienic importance, particularly in relation to the increasing frequency of
sexually transmitted diseases and Aids.

3

The Birth

Confinement at home or in hospital?

This question requires careful consideration, for while the hospital may be well equipped to deal with all kinds of emergencies, it also has dangers and disadvantages which are not present in the home. Because there are so many people in a hospital there is a greater danger of infections such as mastitis (inflammation of the breast), influenza, pemphigus of the newborn, and also now epidemic gastroenteritis, which is the consequence of the indiscriminate use of penicillin and other antibiotics.

The final decision as to where the confinement shall take place is made when the mother is medically examined at the end of the seventh or beginning of the eighth month. The birth will have to be in hospital if the mother's pelvis is too narrow, if a multiple birth is expected, if the child is in an awkward position, or if there are signs of toxaemia or other illnesses in the mother.

If it is not possible to have the baby at home there are a number of points which must influence the choice of hospital. Above all it must be one where the importance of breastfeeding is recognized. In so many places today shortage of or insufficiently trained staff means that the little perseverance needed to establish the mothers' supply of milk is not forthcoming and babies are bottle-fed from the beginning on cow's milk and baby foods. The hospital chosen should also be one where the baby's cot remains beside the mother's bed all the time, only being removed at night if the child is very restless. And finally, the mother must make it clear beforehand that she does not wish the vernix to be washed away when the baby is born. This is the slippery substance covering the baby at birth. (See page 52.)

It is also very important to find out beforehand if it is normal practice in the chosen hospital to given the newborn baby a vitamin K injection, or vaccinate her against TB, and to decide whether one is in favour of this or not (see pages 149–57). In general, immediately after the birth is not the best time to make snap decisions, and sometimes one allows things to happen that one might not have agreed to on more reflection.

The mother's case should be ready packed at least eight weeks before the expected date of birth. It should contain three or more nightdresses which unbutton at the front down to the waist and which can be boiled, a woollen bedjacket, dressing gown, slippers and personal toilet things. Also clothes for the journey home for mother and baby.

For a confinement at home the room where the birth is to take place must be large enough and it is essential that it can be properly heated. Arrangements must be made beforehand to ensure that enough skilled help will be available for mother and baby, so that the baby is not laid aside while the midwife finishes attending to the mother. The midwife or doctor will tell the mother about the various articles she will have to have ready. These will include freshly washed and ironed garments for the child. Ironing is the best way to make laundry sufficiently germ-free.

The father's presence at the birth

Many husbands seem rather helpless and at sea during a woman's pregnancy and feel themselves sidelined. These difficulties are exacerbated if the father is not present at the birth. He may find it difficult to show fatherly feelings to this tiny, fragile being. It is also good for father and mother if they can look back together to this important event, and can later tell the child about it. Additionally one should not underestimate the importance to a couple's relationship of the man standing by the woman in her 'hour of need'.

That is why increasing numbers of men insist on being present at the birth of their child. Doctors and midwives are also happy to allow this now, for the husband's presence frequently has a good effect. In fact some modern obstetrics methods (Lamaze) are even based on the active collaboration of the man. In all events it is important for the father to be sufficiently prepared. He should know something about the physical and emotional processes that occur during contractions, and about the various phases of birth. Relaxation and breathing techniques are something he should practise with his wife beforehand, so that he can really help her during the birth. He must not get over-anxious about the often violent emotional and physical 'storms' unleashed during the last phases of birth. Some midwives even allow the father to cut the umbilical cord and to place the newborn child into the mother's arms.

Painless childbirth

No responsible doctor can promise a woman a completely painless confinement, but it is the duty of the doctor to relieve pain and therefore also the pangs of birth. Dr. Grantly Dick Read's method of natural childbirth (see his books *Natural Childbirth* and *Childbirth without Fear*) can be highly recommended, especially as pain reduction is achieved not by the use of drugs but by the mother's own conscious effort. (Dr. zur Linden would have found the ideas of Professor Leboyer, had he known of them before his death, to be very much in harmony with his own concepts, Ed.)

Any measures to relieve pain which might harm the child should of course be avoided, including hastening or delaying the birth by chemical means. One can regard the hour of birth as a moment of destiny. Sparing a mother any pain whatsoever at delivery may also rob her of a full and powerful experience of the birth. I have seen many mothers who deeply regretted having 'slept through' the birth of their child due to anaesthetic. Nowadays doctors and midwives generally recognize the importance of the mother's 'active' role, and of the part played in combating anxiety of preparation courses prior to confinement. With full knowledge of what is likely to occur, women are more confident and relaxed, and therefore feel less pain.

The beginning of the birth

There are three signs which herald the beginning of the baby's birth: the painless loss of blood and mucous, the painless 'breaking of the waters' which can occur in a sudden flood or just a trickle, and the beginning of labour pains. The latter are caused by contractions of the muscles of the womb and resemble the pains of the monthly period. At first they occur at intervals of 20 to 30 minutes, and when the intervals have decreased to five minutes or less the birth is likely to begin.

Any one of these three signs indicates that the birth is soon to begin, and they can occur in any order. The mother should not wait until all three have manifested. As soon as the first sign occurs she should contact the midwife if the baby is to be born at home, or set in motion the arrangements for her journey to the hospital.

There is no need for fear or anxiety. The new mother will surely manage what countless women have achieved before her and she can have confidence that what is expected of her will be no more than she can bear.

The birth process

During the first stage of labour the cervix and the rest of the birth canal are rhythmically widened to allow the child to pass through. If the mother relaxes and fearlessly allows this to happen quite automatically, she will experience hardly any pain. But if she interferes in nature's work, pain will occur. As Dr Read says: 'Tense woman—tense cervix'. Of course the atmosphere in the room and the mother's relationship with the doctor or midwife should be one of confidence and trust.

When the second stage of labour is reached, the time comes for the mother to take an active part in the bearing-down effort, helping to push the child through the birth canal. This activity gives her great satisfaction and she experiences immense joy at being able to help in her baby's birth. With her help the first part of the child, usually the head, emerges from the birth canal. With the next contraction the body will follow and the child is born. The birth process concludes with the emergence of the afterbirth, which consists of the placenta, the amniotic sheaths and the remainder of the umbilical cord.

4

The Post-natal Period

The first few weeks

Although pregnancy and birth are not illnesses, they do place considerable physical and psychological strain on the mother and she does need time to recover. However long or short her actual time in bed may be (this varies in different countries) she will need a great deal of rest and should sleep whenever she has the opportunity, especially after breastfeeding.

Suitable gymnastics, exercises, massage, and also breast-feeding all help the womb to return to its normal size and the tummy muscles to regain their usual firmness.

Many mothers sleep badly at first. This is a sign of their inner tension. Recognition of this is in many cases all that is required to help the mother become more relaxed and able to enjoy her baby. Weleda sedative teas are also a great help, and often a herbal remedy for stimulating the circulation is the best sleeping draught. Weleda Blackthorn Elixir also helps promote sleep as well as acting as a tonic and stimulating the production of milk. Sleeping tablets should not be taken because the chemical substances they contain are passed on to the baby with the mother's milk.

As a general tonic and also to help prevent thrombosis or inflammation of the veins it is good to take five drops of Arnica D4 with some water three times daily before meals for the first four to six weeks.

Should the newborn baby remain in the same room with the mother?

Apart from very few exceptions, mother and child should not be separated after birth. While the external link between them is cut with the umbilical cord, there are still invisible bonds that are dissolved prematurely if they are unnecessarily separated. The baby's cot should be very close to the mother, so that she can always see him when she wants to. A newborn baby is still very fragile in his physical nature, that is, his individuality is still very loosely connected with his body. Breastfeeding promotes a close contact that draws the baby in to his physical nature.

Many hospitals now acknowledge this and make appropriate arrangements. There is also a further advantage: most women can feel some uncertainty about how to deal with this new, fragile being, especially when it is their first child. If the new mother has the opportunity to observe her child continually, and to ask the doctor, midwife or nurse for advice, she will more easily come to understand and love her child. And she will take more time for her own recuperation. Young women actually often leave the hospital too soon because they do not wish to be continually separated from their child.

Post-natal ailments

After the birth of the baby an open wound is left in the womb which takes a little while to heal. So long as the midwife has been scrupulously clean and done all she should, the mother's own forces of recovery will be sufficient, particularly if she is sensible and has a good quality diet.

Even a cold or mild flu or bronchitis could endanger the mother, and infections like throat inflammations or furunculosis are even more dangerous.

The mother should take her temperature in the morning when she awakes and in the afternoon at about 4 p.m. Taken under the arm it should not exceed 99.5°F (37.5°C). If it rises above 100.4°F (38°C) it could be a sign of incipient mastitis or at least a retention of milk. (It is not certain whether the commencement of lactation causes the temperature to rise as well.) A rise in temperature could also be a sign of trouble in one of the abdominal organs.

Until the wound in the womb has healed entirely, the mother will continue to have a discharge called lochia. This can start to decompose and become rather malodorous. In this case the mother's temperature will rise above 100.4°F (38°C) and she will feel a pressure in the head and general discomfort. The symptoms will be similar if the flow of the lochia becomes congested. Both disturbances can occur during the first eight to ten days after the birth and are easily treated by the doctor who should always be called if there is a rise in temperature.

If the mother's temperature is over 101.3°F (38.5°C) for several days and there are no signs of mastitis or the other ailments mentioned above, she may be found to have infectious childbed fever. If this is so she must be cared for by a private nurse or isolated in hospital so that other women who have just had their babies are not infected. Mother and child may not be nursed by the same person.

Childbed fever usually begins on the third or fourth day after the birth with shivering and a sudden rise in temperature of 104°F (40°C) or more. This could also be a sign of serious mastitis, but whatever is suspected the doctor must be called immediately. Fortunately childbed fever is rare nowadays.

Arnica D4 has already been mentioned as a good tonic and preventative against vein inflammation and embolism. This can be taken from the birth onwards for four to six weeks (5 drops 3 times daily in a little water before meals).

5

The Breastfeeding Period

Diet during breastfeeding

Mother's milk is a complete and perfect organism and its value for the child cannot be stressed too highly. Almost without exception breastfed babies develop harmoniously and without disturbance. Four or five months' breastfeeding provides a basis for good health throughout life. Even the best substitute cannot provide the resistance to diseases given by mother's milk. In view of all this, surely the mother's great wish must be to provide this blessing for her child, while remembering that not only her eating habits but also her state of mind, whether she is worried and anxious or calm and loving, affects the child through breastfeeding.

The nursing mother's diet should be easily digestible and rich in vitamins and minerals and must include sufficient protein. The quality of the food should be as good as possible. The mother must expect anything she eats to be reflected quite soon in her milk and then in her baby.

For instance if the mother has taken some wine, she should not be surprised if her baby falls asleep during his next feed instead of drinking his fill. All stimulants which are toxic for adults also damage the baby via the mother's milk. Alcohol and nicotine should therefore be avoided and great care taken with tea and coffee.

Natural and ordinary foods also contain substances which

pass over into the milk and some of these might disagree with the baby. For instance cabbage eaten by the mother can cause wind and colic in the baby. Some fruit juices, for example pineapple, strawberry, currant, orange, lemon and tomato, when taken by the mother, can cause nappy rash, nettle rash or other rashes in the baby. Even if she eats honey this can cause diarrhoea in the baby. Careful observation will soon show what foods the mother might have to avoid during the breastfeeding period.

Mothers who have to take medicines, especially drugs, must discuss this carefully with their doctor in relation to breastfeeding, and in some cases it might be advisable not to breastfeed. Special mention may be made of sleeping tablets, tranquillizers, antibiotics, sulphonamides, laxatives, steroids and drugs for asthma, heart and circulation.

If meat is desired, it is best to choose the lean white meat of young animals. But protein requirements should be covered mainly with curd cheese (see recipe page 199), cottage and cream cheese and other mild cheeses that do not smell too strong. Since many nursing mothers as well as their babies suffer from wind, it is useful to add caraway seeds to the water when boiling potatoes and other vegetables or to choose a cheese flavoured with caraway. A cup of caraway seed tea is also a help: boil a large pinch of the seeds in enough water for a large cup for 10 to 15 minutes.

Bread is often the cause of flatulence, so choose brands baked with caraway or fennel seeds. Demeter bread and Demeter rusks are also recommended.

Main meals should start with 1 to 3 dessertspoons of grated raw vegetables, especially carrots, possibly mixed with a little cream. It is important, however, that these raw vegetables are grown without the use of chemical fertilizers or insecticides.

Raw fruit is also important, and could alternate with the raw vegetables at the start of the main meals. Or else it is eaten between meals. The evening meal should not be eaten after 6 p.m. or so, since the digestive process slows down over night. Food eaten later remains undigested and weighs on the stomach, pressing on the heart and causing flatulence.

If the mother puts on too much weight, thick soups, puddings and potatoes can be avoided. On the other hand, if she loses weight rapidly she should consult the doctor immediately. It is enough if she weighs herself every two to three weeks.

Beverages will be discussed on pages 50–1.

Menstruation after childbirth

If the mother does not breastfeed her baby she will usually have her first period, a rather heavy one, a month after the birth, and after that her periods will be as usual.

Nursing mothers usually remain without a period until they wean the baby. However, about six or eight weeks after the birth it is quite common for nursing mothers to have one rather heavy period. This is quite normal and gives no cause for concern. The baby will be seen to drink her mother's milk with less relish than usual, but there is no need to stop feeding her because of this.

It is quite possible for a woman to become pregnant again while still breastfeeding. Three or four weeks after the birth a new egg is released from the ovaries ready for fertilization. So even if there is no monthly period during breastfeeding, a new pregnancy is a possibility.

Six or eight weeks after a normal birth the mother should be examined by a gynaecologist so that he can ascertain whether all her abdominal organs have regained their normal size and position. Once this is found to be so, marital intercourse can be resumed.

The technique of breastfeeding

The mother should offer her baby the breast not later than six or eight hours after birth so that she learns to take the nipple and sucks a few times. She will not yet receive much food but this early sucking eases and speeds up the production of milk and when the secretion finally starts it will be less uncomfortable.

During the first few days the mother will feed the baby in bed. She should wash her hands and wipe the nipple with a clean cloth or cotton wool soaked in boiled water. Do not use alcohol or a disinfectant but try to be scrupulously clean without these. The mother lies on her side and relaxes, supported as comfortably as possible by pillows. The baby's nappy is changed and she is then placed with her head level with the nipple. Now the mother grasps the aureola with the fore and middle fingers of her free hand and presses the nipple outwards. The outer hand guides the infant's head so that her mouth touches the nipple. She will instinctively open her mouth and grasp the nipple and part of the aureola so tightly that when she moves her jaw backwards a vacuum forms in her mouth into which the milk flows. The mother should make sure the baby's nose is free for breathing.

This sucking is quite strenuous. During the course of a normal duration of breastfeeding the baby accomplishes it about a million times. It promotes a healthy development of teeth and jaws which is lacking for the most part if the baby only has a bottle teat to suck.

Once the mother is up and about she will need a comfortable chair for feeding, with a footstool high enough to ensure that the baby lying on her knee on a pillow can reach the breast without pulling at it. Her back, arms and legs must be quite relaxed and the baby must be able to lie in a natural position with the arm she is lying on quite comfortable. Both mother and baby must be warm during feeding. The baby can be wrapped in a light shawl and the mother's arms and shoulders should be covered. If the room is quiet and there is nothing to distract her she will concentrate entirely on drinking.

She will take most of her feed during the first three minutes, after which it is good to pause. To detach her the mother may have to hold her nose gently so that she opens her mouth to breathe. She is held upright so that she can more easily bring up the air she has swallowed. It can be a help to pat her gently on the lower half of her back. After several burps she is put to the breast again and allowed to drink till she is satisfied or falls asleep. The milk is more fatty towards the end of the meal but the amount she drinks is far smaller. If she is allowed to suck too long the nipples get sore and this can lead to inflammation.

As soon as she stops drinking heartily or starts playing or going to sleep the meal should be finished. She will then be hungrier at the next meal and will soon develop regular habits without being forced. This should, however, not be done unless she is quite healthy.

If the first breast is empty and the child still hungry, there is no harm in giving her the second. This will probably be quite a regular occurrence in the early weeks and it is a good idea to do it anyway at the evening meal. But the mother must ensure that the breast given first is absolutely empty.

At the end of the meal the baby should again bring up as much wind as possible, otherwise it will disturb her digestion and the pain will make her cry.

And finally the mother should rub the nipples with a few drops of lemon juice. She will find a proper nursing brassiere with disposable pads a great advantage.

Emptying the breast

The baby should not be offered the second breast until the first is absolutely drained. If she is persistently unsatisfied after drinking from a particular breast she should be weighed before and after drinking from that breast to see whether it really contains too little milk.

A breast pump can be used to test whether the first breast is absolutely empty. This is easier but not so effective as milking with the hand, which is best done while seated. The mother takes hold of the breast with both hands, her thumbs uppermost. Stroking the breast with the thumbs from the base towards the nipple she expels the remaining milk. Some women are quite skilled at doing this with only one hand. If there is a lot of milk it can be collected in a sterile container and given to the baby later.

If the first breast is not completely emptied, there is a danger of inflammation with all its undesirable consequences. So the baby must on no account be offered the second breast until the first is empty. If the first breast contains more milk than the baby requires it must likewise be emptied completely with a pump or by milking as described. After each use the pump must be boiled in water with soda and stored in a cloth sterilized by ironing.

The duration of breastfeeding

The most normal and desirable timing is to feed a baby entirely on the breast for five months and then to start gradually weaning till she receives no more breast milk at nine months. Even if the mother still has plenty of milk it is not good to breastfeed for longer than this, as babies who receive only breast milk after nine months can start suffering from anaemia.

Furthermore the point is missed when the next step in loosening the ties between mother and child should take place. This step consists in the baby becoming nutritionally independent of the mother. It is the age when she learns to sit and stand. It is time for her to learn to chew and she can start sitting at table with the family. Nutrition is an 'educational aid' and by this change in feeding habits the baby is taught a certain kind of independence.

It is a mistake to assume that continued breastfeeding will prevent a new pregnancy.

Weaning

Weaning should be done slowly because too rapid a transition to cow's milk can cause digestive disturbances. This is particularly the case if for some reason weaning has to start before the fifth month. It is usually best to avoid weaning during the hottest weeks of the year.

There is not much the mother need do in order to reduce her milk supply. She can drink less and make sure there is no sign of constipation. If despite this she suffers from retention of milk she should apply lukewarm compresses with Weleda Oak Bark Solution (20%) to the breasts morning and evening and wear a firm brassiere.

During the first week of weaning, one meal is replaced by a bottle feed; the second or third meal is usually the best. In the second week a further feed is replaced by a meal of strained vegetables or rusks (preferably Holle Rusks) soaked in milk. It is possible to proceed like this week by week or to take things more slowly, depending on the child and on the schedule of the baby food chosen to replace the breast (see pages 88–94). Great care must be taken in weaning babies who are not quite well, and if there is acute illness this should be cured before weaning starts.

Inability or refusal to breastfeed

There are indeed women who have no milk, but with the majority of those unable to breastfeed the reason lies in mistakes during early attempts which could be easily avoided.

Unfortunately many maternity hospitals still do not do enough to persuade mothers to breastfeed. Often injections given during or after the birth cause insufficient or delayed lactation. Many laxatives and sleeping pills also inhibit lactation directly or else they indirectly affect the child, making her sleepy or giving her diarrhoea so that she does not drink enough. Babies with jaundice of the newborn are also too tired to drink properly.

No doubt there will always be a few women whose vanity prevents them from breastfeeding for fear of damage to their figure. This fear is unfounded if the breasts are treated properly during pregnancy and breastfeeding. Indeed, breastfeeding is positively helpful for the contraction of the abdominal organs. Too little activity and unsuitable brassieres are what make the breast tissues slack. Swimming is a very good regular sport for keeping the tissues firm. Not to breastfeed for egotistic reasons is totally irresponsible. It is even thought that women who have milk but do not breastfeed are more prone to breast cancer in later years.

There are some rare disturbances which make breast-feeding difficult. For instance retracted nipples make it impossible for the baby to take hold and suck. But this condition can for the most part be greatly improved during pregnancy. Several times daily the nipples are sucked out with a breast pump, and wearing nipple shields also helps. In rare cases when they do not improve, the milk can be withdrawn with a breast pump and given to the baby in a bottle. This calls for skill and perseverance but mothers who really know the value of breast milk will gladly undertake the task for several months.

Varying degrees of galactorrhea can occur. In cases where the loss of milk is constant though not great, absorbent pads changed frequently to avoid infection can be used to catch the drips. In serious cases the breast can lose most of its milk.

There are also conditions in which the breasts do not release the milk easily. This is most acute when milk secretion starts very suddenly. It is then necessary to loosen the milk by expelling some either manually or with a breast pump until the breast is less taut.

There are newborn babies who are too weak to suck by themselves, for instance some premature babies. They can be fed on milk obtained from the mother with a breast pump. Indeed, more than any these weak or premature babies need their own mother's milk.

Babies with deformed jaws, for instance a cleft palate, are also unable to suck from the breast and they too can be fed on mother's milk drawn off with a pump. These babies often have a tenacious will to live and they thrive almost without help.

Any noticeable clumsiness in sucking should be pointed out to the paediatrician who should also be consulted if the baby is consistently lazy about drinking.

Sudden shock or excitement can 'make the milk go away'. In fact the milk does not dry up but the ducts are closed by the sudden cramp of shock. In the case of shock the mother should calm down again as quickly as possible, if necessary with the help of 20 drops of valerian tincture in half a glass of sugar water. Any known source of sudden shocks should be avoided, for example television and cinema.

Improving the milk supply

The mother should sleep as much as she can and not do too much physical work if possible. She should drink about two pints (1 litre) over and above what her thirst requires and part of this can consist of three cups daily of Weleda Lactagogue Tea. Apart from its properties of stimulating the milk supply it also has a soothing effect on the digestion of mother and baby and helps combat flatulence in both. However, more than three cups daily can cause diarrhoea in the baby, so the rest of her liquid intake should vary. Milk (buttermilk, sour milk and yogurt), herb teas, grain coffee, fruit juices, elixirs are all suitable, but coffee, ordinary tea (except very occasionally), cola drinks and alcohol are not. Smoking is definitely undesirable for the whole period of breastfeeding.

Weleda also produces a very effective Lactagogue Oil for massaging the breasts several times daily. The resulting increase in milk supply is often astounding. The oil is warming and greatly stimulates the circulation.

Preventing mastitis (inflammation of the breasts)

The mother must always wash her hands thoroughly before feeding and then wash the nipple with plain water. It is good to loosen the milk first by a little gentle massage from the base of the breast towards the nipple. At the end of the feed it is essential to ensure that the breast is absolutely empty before cleaning the nipple with a few drops of lemon juice. The mother must keep her arms warm, specially during feeding.

If a lump appears anywhere in the breast during the feeding period, the breast must be very carefully emptied, if necessary with the help of a breast pump and gentle massage. Then it is lifted firmly with a bandage and if possible the mother should go to bed. If she has a temperature the doctor must be called. Meanwhile a poultice with a thick layer of cool curd cheese is an old remedy for effectively soothing and relieving the pain.

6

The Baby Immediately After Birth

The newborn baby

At last the time comes when the birth has been happily achieved and the newborn baby lies in his mother's arms. Having heard his first cry and made sure that he is really alive, she now experiences in her soul an entirely new feeling of utter happiness. She may touch him, kiss him, look at him, the most beautiful baby in the world, her very own.

As soon as he arrives the baby begins to adjust to his new surroundings, while the first of so many tasks are performed for him. The umbilical cord is cut and he is quickly rinsed with warm water and then carefully dabbed dry with a warmed towel to ensure that the valuable vernix is not damaged. It should be removed only from face and hands.

This fatty, slippery substance, which entirely covers the baby, first helps him slip through the narrow birth canal. That it then also has other uses is becoming increasingly recognized. Apart from fats it contains mineral salts, vitamins and substances akin to protein. Some midwives know that it protects the skin, for they use it themselves to improve their own complexion. It inhibits the germs with which the baby is surrounded in his new environment, it insulates him and keeps him warm, and finally it is a form of nourishment and is absorbed by his skin within a few days. I have frequently observed that if an infant contracts jaundice of the newborn, which can be rather serious, the illness is only slight if he has not had this protective layer removed.

When he is dry he is weighed and measured and then quickly dressed in warmed clothes, placed in his cradle with a hot water bottle (not too hot!) and left in peace to recover from the strains and stresses of being born.

From the moment the umbilical cord is severed, inner changes start taking place which are quite difficult for non-medical people to grasp. These changes are particularly marked during the first few days of life and one can only assist the infant by keeping him warm and absolutely quiet. The warmth of love with which the parents receive him is not enough on its own. He also needs a great deal of physical warmth, particularly in the early weeks.

The severing of the umbilical cord separates the baby physically from his mother. Having received oxygen through his mother's blood he now has to take in with his own lungs the air he will have to share with all of us. He has become our contemporary and fellow citizen.

The baby's first breath brings about a considerable redirection of the blood circulation which before birth bypassed the lungs. Now the wall between the right and the left half of the heart closes and the blood has to circulate through the lungs, refreshing itself there before streaming through the whole body. This very first breath initiates a breaking-down process which is quite prodigious. The embryo has almost twice as many red blood corpuscles as a healthy adult, so within a few hours or days of birth the number of these corpuscles must be halved. Billions of red blood corpuscles perish every minute until the number has decreased from seven or eight million to four million per cubic millimetre.

All these decomposing blood cells have to be dealt with by the digestive organs, particularly the liver. To cope properly the baby needs a great deal of warmth, for of all the organs the liver needs the most warmth. If not kept warm enough the newborn baby might contract serious jaundice which can be dangerous.

An early sign of the breaking-down processes is seen in the activities of the bowel and bladder. First the bowels excrete meconium, a greenish-black substance consisting of thickened digestive juices, uterine fluid swallowed by the baby, cells from the walls of the intestines and fine hair from the embryo's skin. This usually takes three or four days and then the baby starts producing the golden-yellow, sweet-smelling motions of a purely milk diet. During the first few days the baby drinks very little milk and therefore passes water only once or twice a day. Later this happens up to 30 times a day. The first urine passed soon after birth is sometimes reddish in colour due to the salts dissolved in it. This is quite harmless.

The rapid smoothing of the baby's wrinkly skin, the adjustment of the skull bones which are often alarmingly squashed, the starting of metabolism in the mouth, the gullet, the stomach and the intestines, all these are wonderful processes which occur soon after birth. But the most wonderful is the gradual regulating of breath and heartbeat till there are about four heartbeats to every breath. From the very first breath the rhythmical activity of heart and lungs begins, never to cease or tire till the last breath. This is one of the great mysteries of life.

At birth the mucous membranes of the air passages and the intestines are completely sterile, but they are soon well provided with beneficial bacteria. A baby sneezes ten or eleven times a day. This helps clear the nose and is not a sign of a cold unless the sneezing is more frequent.

The newborn infant has only reflex reactions to external stimulation of his sense organs and his movements are without any guidance from the brain. This is interesting since it shows that the limbs can indeed move without any help from brain or spinal cord, though such movement is haphazard and aimless.

Some useful figures

A baby is termed newborn until the external signs of the separation of his organism from that of his mother have been overcome, in particular until the remains of the umbilical cord have dropped off. This happens after 8 to 14 days.

At birth, boys are an average 20 to 21 inches (50 to 54cm) long, girls $\frac{3}{4}$ inch (2cm) less.

Average growth:
in the first month: $1\frac{1}{2}$ to 2 inches (4 to 5cm)
in the second and third months: $1\frac{1}{4}$ inches (3cm) each
in the fourth and fifth months: $\frac{3}{4}$ to $1\frac{1}{4}$ inches (2 to 3cm) each
up to the twelfth month: $\frac{1}{4}$ to $\frac{1}{2}$ inch (1 to 2cm) per month.

At 12 months the average length is $29\frac{1}{2}$ inches (75cm).

At 24 months the average length is 33 inches (85cm).

Normal birth weight is anything between 11 lb (500g) and 4 lb 8 oz (2000g), but babies weighing less than 4 lb 8 oz (2000g) are premature except in the case of twins.

After birth, babies usually lose between 5 and 10 oz (150 to 300g) in weight, but the loss is considerably less if the vernix is not removed from the skin. Then, from the fourth or sixth day onwards, weight is gained again until between the eighth and fifteenth day the birth weight is reached once more. Fairly often this takes considerably longer.

During the first two to three months the daily increase in weight is about $\frac{3}{4}$ oz (20 to 30g). However, some babies gain up to $1\frac{1}{2}$ oz (40g) daily and others as little as just over $\frac{1}{2}$ oz (20g). A well-fed baby doubles his birth weight during the fifth month and trebles it during the eleventh or twelfth month. At the end of the second year his weight will have quadrupled. If the weight at birth was relatively low, the increase will be more rapid.

Breastfed babies and those fed on Holle Baby Food gain weight evenly, while babies fed on other baby mixtures tend to gain in fits and starts. It is quite easy to increase a baby's weight considerably. But the real art of nutrition lies in avoiding any overfeeding. In cases of illness, overweight children are in greater danger than those with the correct weight.

First examination by the doctor

If possible the baby should be examined by the doctor on the first day of his life. For me this is still as happy and exciting a task as it was 40 years ago.

First I look at the general appearance of this new little boy or girl. Is the skin smooth and pink or wrinkled and shrivelled like that of an old person? From this I can tell whether the birth was lengthy or fairly quick, whether it was late or at the right time, and whether the infant will soon need some milk or can wait a while longer. On the first or second day the skin should not yet show any yellowness. At the back of the head or neck and near the eyes many newborn babies have harmless birthmarks which later vanish.

I examine the fine hair which often covers the whole body; I look at the lines in the palms of the hands and on the soles of the feet and at the length of the finger and toe nails. I examine the shape of the whole body and compare the size of the head with that of the chest. Length and weight are the most important measurements for determining the maturity of the newborn. A baby who is too short, underweight, very hairy, has only feeble reactions to external stimuli, i.e. touch and temperature, and one who lacks the sucking reflex is likely to be immature.

Then I examine the head to see whether there are any swellings or whether the bones of the skull, which are still very mobile, are pressed together. I feel the fontanels and the seams between the bones with my fingers. They are not yet fixed or closed, so they can give way to pressure during birth, to any fluctuations of blood pressure in the head, and also accommodate the rapid growth of the brain. The large fontanel is at the top of the head and is the spot where the brain is only protected by some tough skins. Through these one can feel the blood pulsating in the head. The small fontanel is at the back of the head.

The significance of the fontanels is probably much greater than we have realized hitherto. The small one closes soon after birth, but the large fontanel should not be entirely closed until the child is 18 months old. Nowadays certain diets and excessive prescriptions of vitamin D cause the fontanel to close too soon, as early as ten months sometimes. (See pages 127–30).

Then with the help of a spatula or small spoon I examine the cavity of the mouth and palate. Various malformations are possible here which an operation later on can correct, but which meanwhile could cause the child difficulty in sucking.

After this I make sure there is no wry-neck, where the head is drawn to one side by shortened neck muscles. I feel the spine from top to bottom and make sure that all the joints and muscles of the arms and legs work properly and that there are the correct number of fingers and toes.

The state of the navel is examined very carefully. I show the mother how to treat it properly with a sterile dressing fixed in position by a bandage wound round the baby's body starting from below the navel and working upwards, like laying tiles on a roof, to ensure that it will not slip.

Then I listen to the heart with my stethoscope in case there is any congenital abnormality. Normally a newborn baby has 140 heartbeats and about 55 breaths a minute. But soon after birth the heart and lung rhythms have often not yet adjusted themselves. The doctor must then make regular examinations until the adjustment is made, which is usually after about six weeks.

Now the abdomen is examined. I feel the liver, which is normally large at this age, and the size of the spleen is noted. The firmness of the abdominal walls is felt in case there are any weak spots where ruptures might occur. The genitals and the anus are examined.

Finally I look at the visible part of the baby's ears, their shape, size, proportions, angle to the head, the differences between right and left and whether they are delicate or coarse. The external ear reveals a great deal about the physical and soul characteristics of the new human being. Heredity alone cannot explain the infinite variety in the shape of people's ears.

The mother's nerves

A mother with a new baby, especially if it is her first, tends to be far too worried and cramped. In trying to do everything perfectly she easily overreaches herself, becoming more and more ill at ease and losing her inner balance. Fears for the child's health and even his life keep her awake at night; and every time he cries her nerves become more strained. At the same time, during the puerperal period of six to eight weeks, she herself is only gradually recuperating from the strain of the baby's birth.

Usually the mother copes with all this unaccustomed strain for six or seven weeks, but then her nerves give way and she dissolves into tears and despair. She thinks she will never be a capable mother or have enough strength to master her new tasks properly.

However, if she knows there is likely to be this crisis after six or seven weeks she can take precautions in time. Perhaps she has a mother or sister who can help her in the house. She can take more rest, go for regular walks and drink a soothing tea before going to bed (e.g. Weleda Sedative Tea). But above all she must try and become more relaxed in her attitude towards the baby. He will thrive the better if she is at ease and calm.

If she knows these things the new mother will soon be able to laugh at her tears and overcome the crisis in a few days. She should know, however, that when the baby is about three

months old there may be another similar crisis and a further
one sometimes occurs at nine months.

Peace and quiet and the quality of care

The baby is totally unable to protect himself from his surroundings so it is up to the adults around him, particularly his
mother, to select for him the impressions which can help
him. During the very early weeks he should be kept really
quiet, but soon there are many noises which can go on
around him without being harmful. Ordinary household
work and the sound of older brothers and sisters at play and
people talking are noises to which he should soon become
accustomed and which are in no way harmful. But he should
be protected from mechanical noise, even that of the vacuum
cleaner, for as long as possible. Sounds from radio and television are totally alien for him. Music that reaches his ears
indirectly via electrically generated waves is quite unsuitable,
whereas live music, especially singing and lyre playing, is
helpful for the child.

Not only physical noise and bustle or garish lights or cold
but also emotional disturbances, anger, quarrelling or hatred
have direct effects on the child's development.

Adherence to a strict daily rhythm, both in feeding and
general care, greatly helps the baby to establish the regular
functioning of all his organs.

The mother should try not to be too anxious about the
child, for unless she makes a really bad mistake she is not likely
to do him much harm. Sensible caution is quite different from
anxiety. Besides, raising a child requires a certain degree of
faith in God in addition to reliance on one's own intelligence.

After only a few days or weeks the mother will know from the way her baby is crying whether he is thirsty, or whether the trouble is tummy ache or wet nappies. It will also not be long before she can distinguish the crying of her own baby from that of others.

The uniqueness of the baby's cry is one of the first tentative signs of this child's individual human qualities.

The average rate of development

The age at which children learn each new skill is not fixed, so the following timing is only an approximate guide.

First the newborn baby develops all the functions needed for preserving life. Thus nearly every infant learns very quickly how to take the mother's breast and if the child seems in any way clumsy about this the doctor should be consulted immediately. A few hours after birth babies can suck their fingers loudly. Every infant has his own method, beginning even in this activity to show his individuality.

Babies can taste soon after birth and as mother's milk is sweetish their taste is adjusted to sweet things. A bottle-fed baby soon learns to reject a feed which is not sweet enough. The sense of touch develops early, so that babies begin to notice the discomfort of a fold in the nappy or a change of temperature. Soon after birth they can also hear and they jump at sudden noises. Infants only a few days old can react to colours. In the third week the eyes begin to work together, though they do not yet see properly. The pupils contract when light shines on them. But the baby as yet takes no notice of what is going on around him, sleeping most of the time except when feeding.

From the beginning the baby's facial muscles are amazingly mobile and his grimaces endless. The limbs, too, are very mobile, but the muscles are at first in a state of considerable tension, particularly if the child is chilled. In some babies the head is bent rather far back as a result of the position in the womb. The infant can yawn soon after birth and also sneeze, which he does ten or eleven times a day.

In the second month the baby will start to grasp objects if they touch the palm of his hand. At about six weeks he can lift his head when placed on his stomach. He begins to make small noises and babbles gaily, particularly after meals. Sometimes he will follow a close moving object with his eyes and even turn his head. His first smile appears and also his first tears—the newborn infant's crying is tearless.

In the third month he can turn his head when he hears a noise. His eyes can follow light, and moving objects. And he recognizes things he sees often, such as his mother's face which he greets with a smile.

In the fourth and fifth month he begins to grasp purposefully. He lifts his little arm and practises moving first the hand and then the individual fingers, observing this with his eyes. When taken out of his cot he holds his head up and turns it himself, and he sits upright on his mother's arm. While his nappies are being changed he kicks joyfully. He can turn on to his back from his side or even his tummy. When on his tummy he props himself on his arms. He obviously enjoys all his movements.

During the sixth month he learns to place his feet on the floor and straighten his knees as a preliminary to standing. He can sit up alone and thus discovers more and more about his surroundings, recognizing familiar people. He already begins to copy sounds such as clucking noises made with the tongue for his benefit. The room is filled with his joyful chuckling which expresses his good humour and enjoyment of life.

From the seventh to the ninth month all that he has learned so far is perfected. He sits by himself with a straight back on a cushion. He stands holding onto the bars of his playpen and gradually learns to pull himself up on his own. He rolls around his playpen in order to reach his toys. He hardly ceases producing sounds with his mouth, till one day 'mama' or 'dada' is heard for the first time. Fathers of course take it as personal homage if 'dada' is heard first. Whether they are right or not is hard to tell. There are little girls who from the cradle are fascinated by daddy and later by all men! Then the child begins to understand other words, beaming with pleasure for instance when he hears the word 'bottle'. By nine months he should have learnt to chew bread.

Between ten and twelve months he learns to walk to someone calling him if there are enough things to hold on to on the way. He will, however, start being selective, showing sympathy and antipathy clearly towards those around him.

As the child stands and begins to walk at the end of the first year, he now requires freedom to use his limbs and practise as much as possible. Only at night he should be prevented from tumbling about in his bed and ending up completely uncovered.

He eats bread by himself and should begin to drink out of a mug. He sits with his parents at mealtimes, but should not be allowed to taste any titbits from their plates such as cheese or sausage, for this will spoil his taste for his less interesting baby food. He will crawl on all fours, pull himself up on the furniture and walk holding onto it. If led by the hand he will take proper steps. He copies words and sometimes uses them correctly. Children who have been drilled too much will already connect a specific meaning to a word. An eleven and a half month old baby once pointed beaming at the hair on the back of my hand and said 'doggy'.

At 18 months a child has a vocabulary of about 40 words. He should be able to walk and be quite clean and dry during the daytime. Training for this should not start too early. Even nine months is unnecessarily soon, and lengthy potty-sitting often leads to cystitis or other ailments caused by chills.

At two and a half the child can be clean and dry both day and night. This is the time when he also begins to notice himself as an individual for the first time. He no longer feels himself to be a part of his environment but finds that he is a separate person within this environment. Instead of calling himself 'Johnny' he now begins to say 'I', 'I want to have . . .', 'I want to do . . .'

7

Caring for the Baby

The baby's bed

Remembering how protected the baby is in the mother's womb it is obvious that a cot with bars cannot be a very snug place for her once she is born. It is always draughty, however well she is covered. The best bed for the first few weeks is a wickerwork cradle lined with plain pale red or white material. Dots or other patterns are not so suitable. Even a large washing basket will do. This will protect her from draughts and is even a little similar to the womb in shape. The baby needs as much warmth as possible and also protection from all the impressions assailing her in her new surroundings. Therefore a canopy is also necessary. This is best made with pale red silk covered with pale blue silk. Sunlight shining through this makes a wonderfully calming purple glow. Undyed natural silk can also be used. Though blue is a calming colour for adults, small babies are calmed by a beautiful glowing red or better still purple. Light red silk also protects the baby from the fiercer rays of the sun while letting through those which help prevent rickets. So with the protection of the canopy the baby can be allowed much more sunlight than would otherwise be possible.

The mattress should be completely flat, fairly hard and without springs. The best fillings are horsehair or kapok; eelgrass is also quite good. In the olden days mattress stuffing was often of chaff, particularly millet chaff, a warmer and healthier base than many modern mattresses.

A pillow is superfluous but if one is used it should be very thin and of horsehair. This is essential to prevent spinal distortions. Feathers are out of the question because they make the head dangerously hot.

A rubber sheet may be used to protect the mattress but it must be covered with a flannel sheet. Good woollen blankets are the best covering. Cotton is not warm enough and continental quilts are usually too hot and can even be dangerous in hot weather. The blankets can be enclosed in a washable slip with strong tapes at all four corners so that it can be secured under the mattress to ensure that the baby remains covered. When she is older she can be put in a sleeping bag which is also attachable to the four corners of the bed (see pages 79–80).

Rocking the baby

In contrast to most authors on child care I have for many years now been in favour of rocking babies in a cradle.

There is no question of spoiling the child, for only a few minutes of rocking are needed to send her to sleep. The right speed can be found with the help of a lullaby. The rhythmic to and fro resembles breathing in and out and the repeated slight jolt between every swing helps detach the consciousness from the nervous system and send the baby to sleep. The baby can be rocked approximately until she has cut her first teeth, and then she will be ready for an ordinary cot.

It is quite easy to turn a carry cot or basket into a cradle by placing it on a rocking base like that of a rocking horse.

Crying

On the whole a healthy baby with a full tummy and not too wet a nappy does not cry without reason. But some are more restless and cry more readily, for instance if there is a fold in the nappy or if they are bored. These stop as soon as they are attended to. Rudolf Steiner once suggested that a canopy of orange silk might be a help with such children.

At the end of the first month or during the second month, however, there is a period which can last up to four weeks when nearly every baby cries regularly every day for an hour or two and cannot be comforted. So if there is nothing obviously wrong and if the crying takes place at the same time each day, usually towards evening, there is nothing for it but to grit one's teeth and comfort oneself with the knowledge that this is really the baby's first sporting activity which strengthens heart and lungs.

If a baby cries several times a day she usually either has not had enough to drink, which can be difficult to determine with breastfed babies, or she has a pain, perhaps caused by wind. A little fennel tea will usually comfort her. Boil 1 level teaspoon of fennel seeds in 1 cup of water for 1–3 minutes. Add a little sugar to taste. Some aniseed can be boiled with the fennel if wind is the trouble. Also her mother can pick her up and carry her a little with her head face down in the crook of the arm and her warm hand supporting the baby's tummy while she gently pats her behind with the other hand. Then if she has a cradle she can rock the baby for a few minutes, or if not then rock her in her arms.

Weak babies or the babies of older parents are sometimes too quiet and do not cry even if they are hungry.

Nearly all babies cry after feeding until they have brought up swallowed wind (see page 45).

Keeping the baby's abdomen warm

On the whole babies are not kept warm enough nowadays. Except on the hottest days it is hardly possible to keep a baby too warm during the early months.

The abdomen, in particular, must be kept warm at all times. Chills caught in that region during nappy changing are the most frequent cause of discomfort, pains and hiccups (see below).

The damp warmth inside the nappy usually has a temperature of about 98.6°F (37°C) while room temperature is often not more than 65° to 68°F (18° to 20°C). The evaporation caused by this drop of 30 or more degrees F (19°C) is a great shock to the system and often results in colic pains or bladder chills and worse. Spring and autumn are the most difficult seasons.

So the room should be as warm as possible when the baby is to be changed. In addition, when the nappy is partly undone it is a good idea to dry underneath it with a towel before opening it completely. Keep the abdomen covered all the time, use warm water and work quickly. The clean nappies should be warmed. The best way is to keep the next lot of nappies and a change of clothes with the baby in her cot.

Hiccups

A baby who often suffers from lengthy bouts of hiccups, a cramp of the diaphragm, is being treated wrongly in some way. Either her abdomen has been chilled during nappy changing (see above), or her bottle has not been warm enough. When feeding with the bottle it is important to keep it warm with a woollen cover or to warm it up every few minutes in hot water.

The ancient Greek doctor Hippocrates recommended tickling in the nose with a feather as a cure for hiccups. Sneezing stretches the diaphragm and this brings the hiccups to an end. A warm camomile bag laid on the tummy usually does the trick too. Fill a small muslin bag with camomile flowers and heat on the lid of a boiling saucepan. Then place on the baby's tummy.

The dummy (pacifier)

Babies who do not want to suck a great deal should use their fingers. But if a good deal of sucking is done a suitable dummy should be provided because the danger of deforming the gums is too great. This is not only ugly but can affect health. Enormous numbers of children have to undergo corrective treatment after spoiling their gums or teeth by sucking fingers or thumbs. The best dummy is one which causes the baby or small child to suck as she would at the mother's breast. 'NUK-Sauger' dummies made in Germany are excellent if obtainable.

While teething, a baby can wear a necklace of amber beads on which she can bite. A single piece of amber on a ribbon or a ring of ivory or horn, but not plastic, is also good, as is the traditional orrisroot. Dummy sucking should cease no later than the change of teeth.

Should the baby lie mostly on her tummy?

This is frequently recommended, but the reasons given are unconvincing. They seem to stem more than anything from the general tendency to equate human beings with animals. Because dogs and cats lie on their bellies does not mean that this is the best or most 'natural' position for human babies. Indeed, it is more in keeping with human dignity not to lie facing the earth, and down the centuries babies have thrived quite happily lying on their backs facing the universe or lying on one or other side. Similarly, the baby is the only creature on earth who can look into her mother's face when being fed. Fortunately, science is at last coming to realize that right from the moment of conception the human being is human and not animal. More recently some findings suggest that lying on the tummy may be implicated in cot death.

Sunbathing

Essential though the rays of the sun are for the baby, it can be very harmful to expose her to them too early or too directly, but there are of course seasons and places with little sunshine which make it necessary to be more generous. The skin should be allowed to tan only slowly. From three or four months onwards in good weather the sun can be allowed to shine on the naked baby's back and tummy for a few minutes, but the head must always be protected. It has been discovered that blue sky is just as effective as direct sunlight.

Daily fresh air

As with everything, a happy medium must be found here. Any attempt to toughen the child can lead merely to a hardening and a dulling of the senses whereas the aim should be to maintain a healthy sensitivity to external stimuli provided for instance by sun, air, water and food. So there should be no enforced exposure, for instance to cold wind.

After the sixth week the baby should have some fresh air daily. At first her cot can be placed by the open window and then when the weather is good her pram can be left for many hours on the balcony or in the veranda or garden so long as her head is protected from wind and sun. This is much better than taking her for a walk in the pram. In town the latter should be avoided as long as possible. The noise of cars rushing past shocks the baby and the worst exhaust fumes lie low on the road at the level of many prams. There is much to be said for prams on high wheels so long as the baby is firmly strapped in once she can sit up.

It is equally pointless to take her for a walk in a pram which is completely sealed against the elements. One might as well spare her the jolting.

Babies cool very quickly in a cold wind, so in windy weather their time out of doors must be correspondingly shorter. East winds and cold below 21°F (minus 4°C) call for particular caution, extra clothes and coverings, and even a hot water bottle.

Infant gymnastics

Anyone who has observed attentively how babies practise with their little fists, how they watch intently as the fingers open and close and the hand turns in every direction, knows that this is one of the most touching and intimate manifestations of the coming together of body and soul.

And anyone who has also seen an infant gymnast at work, bending and stretching the little limbs backwards and forwards like parts of a machine in a tempo and rhythm quite foreign to the child must realize that this is utter madness and even a crime against the child.

Justifying this sort of thing by saying that the babies enjoy it is a dangerous conclusion. Within a few days the infant's healthy instincts can be ruined. Gymnastics at this age start a development which is just as 'good' as the blossoming of a plant in a hothouse. The damage shows years later in weaknesses of the motor system which has been stimulated too early and too unnaturally.

It is quite another matter if the mother gently and playfully stimulates the baby to use her limbs. She can let the baby push against her hand with her feet or she can place her on her tummy and encourage her to turn her head. This kind of gentle activity can never be harmful.

Care of skin and hair

The newborn baby's skin is red and usually very sensitive and easily inflamed, particularly during the early weeks.

Except for the first quick rinse after birth the baby should not be bathed until the navel is completely healed and dry. Washing with lukewarm water and a little baby soap is quite sufficient. The soaps, creams, oils and powders used for the baby should be the purest obtainable and perfumed only by natural ingredients. A special flannel and separate water should be used for the face. If the baby has hair this need not be washed daily. Cotton wool or soft tissues are best for cleaning eyes, nose and ears.

Around the large fontanel babies with hair often have a fatty secretion which takes the form of a greyish scaling. This is quite harmless and without endangering the fontanel it can be softened with oil and then gently scraped off with a comb or a card.

The protective coating of oil in the baby's skin can be enhanced with the application of a pure vegetable oil once a week, any surplus being removed with a towel. This is particularly beneficial for weak babies who feel the cold easily. Weleda Hypericum Oil is very good.

Those parts of the skin which are constantly in contact with wet and dirty nappies may need protecting with oil or cream.

The baby's hair can be brushed with a soft brush with natural bristles. A brush which is too hard stimulates the secretion of oil. There is no danger of damaging the fontanel with gentle brushing or combing.

Nappies

Since a baby wets her nappy up to 30 times a day it is impossible to change her every time. She should be changed before every meal and once or twice in between if she cries to show that she is uncomfortable. This applies to the night as well, but one or at the most two changes will do at night if she does not cry. Most babies produce a dirty nappy up to three times a day and when this happens they should be changed immediately. Usually mothers will find themselves changing nappies about seven times a day at first. They should develop the skill of accomplishing this quickly and without disturbing the baby.

Whatever nappies are used, the final result of the nappy procedure should be a firm bundle, especially in the first three months. A shawl wrapped neatly round everything else is a good way of achieving this. If possible wait till the baby is older before using disposable nappies.

Disposable nappies are practical and hygienic on short journeys, but longer use may lead to changes in the skin bacteria environment due to chemical treatment of nappies. Disposables do not wrap a baby in the same quality of living, loving warmth that a natural material has, although they are of course a help to a busy and perhaps stressed mother. If disposables are used, try to ensure that they have not been chemically treated. They are, in addition of course, a burden for the environment, both during production and in disposal.

Plastic pants are very undesirable. They cause overheating of the abdomen which leads to an even greater risk of chill when the nappies are changed. They also probably cause certain components of the urine to be absorbed by the skin. Many babies get sore when plastic pants are used. If it is impossible to manage without, a plastic square which does not make the nappy bundle airtight can be used.

Bathing

Daily bathing is undesirable, especially when it means the daily use of soap. The baby's bottom is washed several times a day anyway and the rest of her is not likely to get too dirty.

Apart from the fact that bathing is very strenuous for many babies, soap deprives the skin of the valuable oils which help keep her warm and protect her from infection and various external irritations. It cannot be replaced by even the finest oil applied externally. When oil is used on the baby's skin it should be vegetable oil and definitely not mineral or tar-based.

Bathing should always take place before a meal, never after. In winter twice and in summer three times a week is quite sufficient. After the first few months, well-covered babies can be bathed more often. The temperature of the water should be 97°F (36°C) and the room at least 68°F (20°C). The best way to ascertain the correct water temperature is by using the elbow. The baby should not be in the water for more than five minutes. Since windows and doors should remain closed, everything must be prepared in advance and placed within reach of the mother's free hand: water thermometer, bowl of lukewarm water for the face, flannel for the face, flannel for the rest, cotton wool, container for used cotton wool, baby soap, baby powder, baby cream, oil, towel, clean clothes, hairbrush and comb.

Start with the face (do not submerge the ears) and finish with the bottom. With girls sponge from the front backwards between the legs to prevent bacteria from entering the vagina. After the bath dry the baby very carefully all over, in all the folds and the palms of the hands. With girls part the lips of the vagina and wipe carefully from front to back with cotton wool soaked in oil. Powder lightly in all folds, under arms and between legs.

Sleep

The baby's sleep should be regarded as sacrosanct. Never wake her if at all possible, but if once in a while it is necessary then do so very gently. Some babies look very pale while asleep.

During the early weeks babies sleep nearly all day except while being fed and changed. Only hunger, thirst and the discomfort of dirty nappies wake them and they often fall asleep before they have finished a meal.

The regular crying time described earlier (see page 67) falls in the second month, but otherwise the baby still sleeps nearly all the time.

During the third month the baby lies awake for some of the time playing with her hands, kicking with her legs and practising her first sounds. This continues, but by the sixth month she should still be sleeping for 12 to 14 hours at night and for two or more hours morning and afternoon.

At one year and more she should still sleep 12 hours at night and also some time during the morning and afternoon.

Every hour of sleep is useful for the child and her development. It should be possible to do ordinary housework and even put on the light without disturbing a good sleeper. Overfed babies and nervously excitable babies usually sleep less than they should.

Swallowing air

If the baby cries for a long time and seems to be in pain, check whether her tummy is swollen and hard with wind. Babies often swallow air with their food and this stretches the stomach, pushing up the diaphragm. This interferes considerably with breathing and the functioning of the heart and can be most painful. If the baby has to breathe through her mouth because her nose is blocked with a cold she is more likely to swallow air while feeding. Quite often a drink of just over an ounce (30g) of caraway seed tea will help. (Boil a large pinch of caraway seeds in enough water for a large cup for 15 minutes.) This diminishes the effect of the wind but it may not help sufficiently. The doctor may have to release it by inserting a thin tube into the baby's stomach. About an ounce (30g) of fennel or aniseed tea (see page 67) helps with very young babies, combined with a camomile compress round the abdomen (see page 69.)

Colds

If the baby has a cold and a blocked nose she will keep trying to suck and then let go to breathe till she gives up, crying with frustration. Her nose can be cleared with a weak solution of salt in water inserted into the nostrils on a blob of cotton wool. Dissolve just over $\frac{1}{4}$ oz (9g) of salt in two pints (1 litre) boiled water. If necessary follow this with a little Weleda Catarrh Cream inside and outside the nose.

No one with a cold or flu should be allowed near a small baby. If the mother herself has a cold she should wash her hands very carefully before attending to her and if possible cover her own mouth and nose with a mask or muslin nappy.

Bowel movements

During the first five or six days the bowel excretes meconium, a greenish black substance. After a few days its place is taken by the golden-yellow, pleasantly fragrant motions of a purely milk diet. At first there may be up to six motions a day, some of which may be rather liquid or bitty. The motions of a bottle-fed baby are usually greyish yellow in colour, rather firm and stale smelling. After the first week, the baby does not usually pass more than one or two motions in 24 hours.

With breastfed babies, there is no cause for worry if several days pass without a motion, so long as the baby has no tummy pain. The cause may be an insufficient intake of milk, so it is sensible to weigh the baby before and after meals to check the amount she is taking.

Clothes for the baby and small child

As adults we know how uncomfortable it is to feel cold and how it prevents us from working properly either physically or mentally. A baby feels even more uncomfortable and yet she cannot complain verbally. If her mother is observant she will notice what is the matter if the baby is too pale or if there are disturbances in her development. The soul and spirit need sufficient warmth for their work of moulding and remoulding the body. What is said in this section applies particularly to the first three years.

As far as possible all the baby's clothes should be made of natural materials such as wool, cotton and silk. Synthetic fibres are a very poor substitute.

The baby's vests should be of wool or pure silk. Cotton and linen are not warm enough, particularly for delicate babies without enough fat. A thin woollen vest is the baby's most important item of clothing. So long as it is clean it should be kept on at night.

All fresh clothes should be warmed before they are put on,

particularly in winter. A good way is to keep them in the cot with the baby as mentioned above. Otherwise every change of clothing brings about a considerable loss of heat.

However, it must be emphasized that on hot summer days there can be a danger of overheating which can lead to serious diarrhoea. Signs of this are restlessness, a red face and sweaty hair. Therefore let it be said once again that woollen blankets should be used since they allow for ventilation, whereas quilts can retain too much heat (see page 66).

While the baby is wrapped in a fairly firm bundle for the first three months (see section on nappies, pages 73–4), at about four months she can start wearing rompers or leggings and is allowed to kick for a few hours each day. But at night she should still be wrapped fairly firmly, though of course never so tightly that she cannot move her legs at all. It seems that the baby needs a fairly firm wrapping until the development of her internal organs has reached a certain stage. This does not mean that she should not be allowed to kick while she is being changed or bathed. As with everything one must find the golden mean. Experience has shown that if the limbs are left too free too early there is a tendency later for scatter-brained lack of concentration, while if they are swaddled too tightly there is a tendency for physical and mental inhibition and clumsiness. As has been said, the soul and spirit work their way into the body and are affected by what they experience in the limbs at this early age.

Towards the end of the first year, when the baby begins to stand, it is time to give her limbs all the freedom they want so that she can learn to use them. But at night she should still be prevented from tossing and turning too much. The continental idea of a warm sack for the body and legs attached to a bodice which leaves the arms free is a very good solution. Tapes attached to the bottom of the sack and to the bodice are fixed under the mattress tightly enough to prevent the child from standing up but slack enough to allow her to turn over. In this way she cannot kick off her bedclothes and catch a chill. The sack has a zip down one side to allow for nappy changing.

When the baby starts to crawl the clothes must be designed to prevent her from catching a chill in the lower part of the body. Heat rises, so the floor is the coldest and draughtiest part of most rooms. Small girls in particular often contract an inflammation of the bladder or worse while they are learning to crawl. They should wear woolly pants, tights and trousers.

The general rule is that the lower part of the body must always be kept warm while the upper part can be exposed much more to the fresh air. The tummy is the kitchen of the body where the cooking (digestion) takes place. To do its work the liver, the most important digestive organ, needs the considerable heat of 102.2° to 105.8°F (39° to 41°C). The child does not have enough strength to create this warmth if her abdomen is not sufficiently clothed. The mother should therefore not be surprised if the baby has no appetite, is pale and does not develop properly.

If children wear ankle socks or knee socks their knees and thighs will be far too cold and the chill creeping up towards the abdomen affects not only the work of bladder and liver but also interferes with the development of all the abdominal organs. The consequences in later life are far more serious than most mothers imagine.

A child's foot usually looks completely flat until the third or fourth year because the arch is filled with a cushion of fat which remains until the muscles of the foot are strong enough to carry the weight of the child. The development of the muscles is hindered if the child wears boots or shoes with special supports or soles. So buy good shoes with flexible soles or good sandals. And avoid the X-ray apparatus still used in some shops. They can damage the cells in the growing foot, though the consequences do not appear for many years.

Dangers due to carelessness

- Anything pointed is dangerous. Safety pins should only be used if they are so large that even the strongest baby cannot open them.
- Toys with wooden balls or beads should only be given if the balls and beads are too big to be put in the mouth. Mind that older children do not give the baby conkers or marbles! First aid if something is swallowed: Place the baby on her tummy, support her head and hold her nose so that she open her mouth. Pat sharply with the flat of the hand on the upper part of the back. If something sharp or spiky is swallowed, feed the baby immediately with semolina pudding or mashed potato and call the doctor!
  If an object is blocking the windpipe (the child turns blue!), place a hand on either side of the chest and press sharply. The expelled air will remove the object.
- Care should be taken with bedding. A child can smother herself with a feather pillow. After the third month a baby is safest in a sleeping bag as described on page 80.
- Plastic bags are a menace. Children can pull them over mouth and nose, and suffocate.
- Babies have been known to strangle themselves with the

ribbon to which their dummy is attached. Any ribbons or cords (e.g. on toys or curtains) near the baby are dangerous.

- Babies should not be given any breakable toys, particularly plastic animals, dolls or rattles.
- All toys must be washable and the paint non-poisonous.
- Babies should not be left alone with animals. It happens again and again that cats sit on babies and smother them. Dogs must not be allowed to lick the baby.
- People with colds or flu should not be allowed near the baby. If the mother has a cold she can tie a nappy round mouth and nose while attending to the baby. She should also wash her hands thoroughly.
- Babies and children should never travel in the front seat of a car. In an accident they are far safer on the back seat.

8

Feeding the Baby

1. BREASTFEEDING

Feeding times

Until there is enough milk, no fixed rhythm of feeding is adhered to, but feeding should be on demand. Then a rhythm of feeding every four to four and a half hours gradually develops. One starts in the morning with the breast which has a stronger flow of milk, and feeds until the child is full, giving the other breast as well.

According to old tradition babies were fed at around the following times: 6 a.m., 10 a.m., 2 p.m., 6 p.m. and 10 p.m.; and to begin with at 2 a.m. as well. This regular sucking every four hours helps stimulate the supply of milk.

It is a good idea to try to adhere to fairly uniform intervals between feeds since the stomach needs time to digest and recover. One should gradually accustom the child to this rhythm and not react too swiftly if he cries. The restlessness caused by this can be bad for both mother and child. Continually changing feeding times is, in the long-term, harder on the nerves than a few days' effort to establish a clear rhythm.

While regularity and a clear pattern are good for breast-feeding, it would be wrong to insist that the child drinks the same amount at each feed. There is no need to weigh a healthy child after every feed.

On the first day the baby can be put to the breast twice but will obtain only a few drops. If the birth was lengthy and the baby is rather dried out with a very wrinkly skin, he can be given a few drops of fennel or camomile tea with a pipette or tiny spoon but he will probably take less than $\frac{1}{3}$ oz (10g). The tea can be slightly sweetened.

Proper feeding begins on the second day. The baby is put to the breast six times, though very placid babies who were heavy at birth are usually satisfied with five meals from the start. Given six meals, the amount required will be $\frac{1}{3}$ to $\frac{2}{3}$ oz (10 to 20g) and given five meals up to 1 oz or just over (30g). During these early days the baby obtains only the colostrum, a thick yellow liquid, so if there is not enough he can be given a little camomile or fennel tea with a spoon. The colostrum is extremely valuable for the baby and he should have every available drop.

On the third day the amount needed will be six times nearly 1 oz (25g) or five times just over 1 oz (30g).

On the fourth day the amount is increased by under $\frac{1}{4}$ oz (5g) per meal. By the fifth and sixth day the milk supply starts to be properly established and the baby will need six times about $1\frac{3}{4}$ oz (50g) or five times just over 2 oz (60g).

From the seventh day the amount will increase by about 10g per meal each day. But there are no exact rules and every baby has his own individual needs.

The following rule of thumb may be helpful for calculating the amounts needed in the early weeks.

Up to and including the sixth week the amount of breast milk taken daily should be about one sixth of the baby's weight. For example if the baby weighs 8 lb (3600g), the daily amount would be 8 (3600) ÷ 6 = 21 oz approx (600g) or $4\frac{1}{4}$ oz (120g) for each of five feeds. From the seventh week onwards the baby should take one seventh of his weight. For example if he weighs $10\frac{3}{4}$ lb (4900g) the daily amount would be $10\frac{3}{4}$ (4900) $\div$ 7 = $1\frac{1}{2}$ lb (700g), i.e. 5 oz (140g) for each of five feeds.

Some babies are exceptionally large and they do need more. However, if given a few teaspoons of unsweetened fennel tea before each meal they will drink less greedily and not exceed the normal amount so easily.

Some breastfed babies begin to sleep through the 10 p.m. feed at four or five months and take more in the morning instead. The daily intake of these babies is then somewhat less than it would be with five meals, though they then usually drink more than 7 oz (200g) at each feed.

To check the amount taken at a particular feed, weigh the baby with all his clothes before and after feeding; and add up the total for the daily intake. If he is not getting enough, do not immediately try to supplement the breast with cow's milk. Instead try to satisfy him with a little herb tea or diluted fruit juice. He will then be hungrier for the next meal and will suck harder, thus increasing the milk supply.

During the early weeks there is no reason why the baby should not be given a little drink during the night if he is thirsty. Give him only a small amount of sweetened herb tea and he will soon get into the habit of sleeping through the night, since it will not be 'worth his while' to make a big fuss for nothing but a little tea. If he does not fall asleep again after he has been changed and given $\frac{2}{3}$ to 1 oz (20–25g) of herb tea, it may be presumed that he is not receiving sufficient nourishment during the day, so he must be given more at the 10 p.m. feed or at each feed during the day.

A sixth daily feed is necessary for delicate babies who cannot take too much food at once and also for strong, hungry babies. There is no need to let hungry babies cry for hours at night, and after a short time, four to six weeks, babies often sleep through the night of their own accord. If the baby does wake at night it is essential to change his wet or dirty nappies.

No later than the eighth week even completely breastfed babies should begin to have additional foods. A start can be made with a few teaspoons of carrot juice or small amounts of fruit puree. If these agree with the baby, the amount can be increased to twice 1 oz (30g) daily. From the twelfth week, the carrot juice can be replaced by mashed carrot.

During the fourth month the fruit puree can be mixed with rusk, or raw grated apple mixed with mashed banana can be given. Thus during the fifth and sixth month a breastfed baby will be having four feeds from the breast and in addition a mid-morning feed with mashed vegetable and an afternoon feed with fruit puree.

What if the baby refuses the breast?

Some newborn babies, especially those who are premature, are too weak to suck. They can be fed on milk obtained from the mother with a breast pump. Indeed, more than any, these weak or premature babies need their own mother's milk.

Babies with deformed jaws, for instance a cleft palate, are also unable to suck from the breast and they too can be fed on mother's milk drawn off with a pump. These babies often have a tenacious will to live and thrive almost without help.

Any noticeable clumsiness in sucking should be pointed

out to the doctor, who should also be consulted if the baby is consistently lazy about drinking.

If the baby has once or twice been given a bottle with too large a hole in the teat he may refuse the breast because it demands more hard work. Or if he has a cold and a blocked nose he will keep trying to suck and then let go to breathe. (See *Chills*, page 139.)

The baby may also refuse the breast if he and his mother are both too nervous and excitable. The mother will have to try to be more calm and take life more slowly, and the doctor may have to help with a harmless sedative or a calming herb tea. With patience this situation can usually be overcome and the baby still be persuaded to drink from the breast.

2. BOTTLE FEEDING

It is quite easy to increase a baby's weight considerably. But the real art of nutrition lies in avoiding any overfeeding. In cases of illness, overweight children are in greater danger than those of the correct weight.

What are biodynamic foods (Demeter)?

The realization that modern agricultural methods were aimed one-sidedly at increasing the *quantity* of food available for the ever-growing population of the earth, while *quality* was deteriorating alarmingly, led a number of farmers and gardeners to seek advice from Rudolf Steiner on how to care for soil, crops and livestock in ways that would increase their health and quality rather than their quantity only. From these meetings the biodynamic method of agriculture and horticulture evolved, in which special attention is paid to the preparation of natural fertilizers and composts.

Grain, vegetables and fruit grown in accordance with these methods are of the highest quality. Doctors who have been advising their patients for years to use such produce know the beneficial effect on health and growth, while anyone eating them cannot fail to notice their superior flavour and quality. Recognized producers use the brand name 'Demeter'. This, and similar products under other names are available in health food shops.

Feeding with Demeter Holle Baby Food

This baby food is made from grain grown by the biodynamic method. After 40 years' experience I can say without hesitation that its use with cow's milk guarantees the best possible development in babies. They drink, and later eat it with obvious relish and their development shows that it is the best possible substitute for breast milk.

It is simple to use, but the following suggestions will enable mothers to exercise their responsibility and ingenuity with a degree of variation not possible with ordinary baby foods. In this way they can really enter into the way in which they feed their babies, and need take nothing for granted.

The number and timing of feeds and the amount per feed

On the whole the baby can be given as much as he takes eagerly. Amazingly, when the food conforms to mother's milk as closely as possible, babies usually take to within 5g the amount they would have taken if fed at the breast. It is not necessary for the baby to drink exactly the same amount at each feed. But though it is good to be flexible about the amount, it is necessary to be quite strict about the number of meals and their timing. Demand feeding has its place only in the early days until the baby has found his own rhythm. It is a great help to the little organism if the feeds are given regularly at the same time and with the same intervals each day. This is particularly so with babies who are not breastfed. During the early weeks, once a rhythm has been established, the baby will wake almost to the minute at the right time for each feed. The mother will know that if he cries at other times there is something else the matter.

FOR THE PREPARATION OF THE MILK AND HOLLE CEREAL MIXTURE SEE APPENDIX THREE, PAGE 197

Bottle feeding during the first month

On the first day give only a few teaspoons of fennel tea. Proper feeding starts on the second day with five feeds of about $\frac{2}{3}$ oz (20g) of milk and water (half and half).

On the third day feeding with the Holle mixture begins. However, in the case of babies weighing less than $6\frac{1}{2}$ lb (3000g) at birth and those who are not very robust, it is best to start with Demeter (biodynamic) wheat or oat flakes in place of the Holle No. 1 mixture for the first four weeks, and to change to Holle No. 1 in the fifth week. (Holle No. 2 can be started in about the fourth month.)

Average babies are offered five feeds of about 1 oz (25 to 30g) of Holle No. 1 mixture on the third day. After this a daily increase of up to $\frac{1}{3}$ oz (5 to 10g) per feed continues till the tenth day, when five feeds of about 3 oz (80g) each are given.

From the end of the second week the amounts given on pages 84–5 for breastfeeding apply, with the exception of premature or otherwise ailing babies.

Bottle feeding during the second month

If the baby's mixture has so far been with Demeter oats or wheat flakes, now is the time for the changeover to a mixture made with Holle Baby Food No. 1, which is made from biodynamically grown oats, wheat and rye made easily digestible by a special process. Many babies already thrive on this mixture during the first month, but it is too heavy for some to start with (see above).

Bottle feeding during the third month

The amount given can be increased gradually, but should not exceed 28 oz (800g) daily for an average baby. At the same time the transition can be made from the half-and-half Holle No. 1 mixture to the two-thirds Holle No. 1 mixture (see Appendix Three, p. 197) by giving the thicker mixture for an additional feed every two days until all the feeds are made with this. If sufficient weight increase is not achieved with 28 oz (800g) per day, the amounts for the fourth month can be given towards the end of the third month.

By the end of the third month the baby will be having four or five bottle feeds. In addition he may have small amounts of mashed raw fruit, particularly grated apple, and also carrot juice and Weleda or Wala elixirs of wild fruits (Cranberry, Blackthorn, Rowan, Rose Hip).

Bottle feeding during the fourth month

The changeover to Holle Baby Food No. 2 can now begin and like all changes in diet it should take place slowly. First the new mixture is used for one feed only. Two days later a second feed is changed over, and so on until all feeds are of Baby Food No. 2, which is a wholegrain food. After this the amount of milk can also be increased until the daily amount is about 21 oz (600g) milk and 14 oz (400g) Baby Food No. 2, slightly sweetened with sugar, divided into five feeds of $6\frac{1}{2}$ to 7 oz (180 to 200g) each.

Average babies change over to four meals a day during the fourth month and start on more solid food. A typical day's meal would be: 6–7 a.m. a two thirds mixture of Baby Food No. 2; 11 a.m. increasing amounts of vegetables (organic or biodynamic carrots or spinach), followed by a bottle of Baby Food No. 2, two thirds mixture (7 oz or 200g if the baby is having four meals a day); during the afternoon, 3 p.m., increasing amounts of mashed fruit followed again by a bottle of Baby Food No. 2; in the evening, 6 p.m. repeat of the morning feed, or start to give a pap made from Baby Food No. 2.

Feeding during the fifth month

The milky meals remain as for the fourth month. The afternoon meal can be augmented by mashing two rusks with the stewed fruit. The midday vegetable feed is also increased to a proper meal. If the baby refuses vegetables, mix them with some fruit.

There is no need to worry about overeating. Hardly any child of this age will eat more than eight to ten dessertspoons of mixed vegetables and fruit.

In winter and spring several dessertspoons of fresh fruit juice may be added to the vegetable mixture immediately before feeding, but remember that fast electric mixers and also simple exposure to air destroy vitamins.

Most babies will now be having four meals a day, so that the last meal can be at 8 p.m. or sooner. The longer sleep during the night partly replaces nourishment, so that the bottle feeds need only be increased by about 1 oz (20 to 30g).

Feeding from the sixth to the ninth month

The child now starts to need more and more solid food. Bottle feeds can be reduced to two a day, or from the eighth month one bottle feed in the morning and a milky pudding in the evening. During the eighth month, the transition can be made from two thirds milk to undiluted milk for the mixture. One of the meals now consists entirely of vegetables and another of a mixture of mashed fruit and rusk. Each meal is about 7 oz (200g). The vegetables are also mixed with grain products, e.g. flakes of various kinds. Some butter may be added, or a little unheated oil, and possibly a pinch of sugar.

If the child is thirsty, specially during the summer, give him weak fennel, camomile or yarrow tea.

Extra fruit should be given before the meal, especially before the milk pudding. Thus the evening meal can consist of fruit followed by the milk pudding, or milk pudding mixed with rusk or curd cheese. The child can be given a biscuit, rusk or crust of wholemeal bread to nibble at by himself.

Suitable vegetables are organically or biodynamically grown carrots, spinach, cooked lettuce, young kohlrabi, cauliflower and tomatoes. This makes considerable variety possible. The choice of vegetables and grains should depend on the nature of the individual child.

(See *Some considerations when choosing food*, pages 98–9.)

Feeding from the tenth to the twelfth month

By about the ninth month many children already have two or more teeth, but whether they have teeth or not, now is the time for them to learn to chew. If the gums are very sore with teething then wait a little, but otherwise start giving small cubes of bread with butter and honey or some good jam. The further development of the jaws and also the maintenance of healthy teeth have a great deal to do with sufficient chewing. So from this age and continuing right through childhood it is good to ensure that children do enough proper chewing by giving them every day a thick piece or crust of hard, stale wholegrain bread which demands strenuous chewing.

Milk can now be given undiluted, but it is still more digestible if it is diluted, perhaps with a little grain coffee. The daily amount should still not exceed about 500g.

The child can of course now join the family at table for some or all meals, but he should not yet share the adults' diet, which is still too rich in protein. Once he has tasted eggs, meat and sausage he will start refusing his own more suitable but less interesting diet.

Curd cheese thinned with a little milk and mixed with any fruit in season is an excellent dish for the child's evening meal. Care should be taken to ensure that the cheese is of good quality. Alternatives are semolina pudding with fruit or rusks soaked in fruit juice. Up to 200 or 300g should satisfy the child.

3. MILK-FREE DIET FOR BABIES

A mother whose baby is allergic to cow's milk and who herself has insufficient breast milk is faced with a considerable problem, especially if her doctor sees no way round starting the child too early on meat and eggs as an alternative. Many mothers will feel instinctively that this is not the solution.

A homoeopathic preparation made by Weleda from potentized cow's milk is now available. It is found that the allergy often disappears after a single dose of a few drops, provided that it is a genuine milk allergy. In the case of an allergy to the mother's milk, the preparation can be made from her milk, even if she herself is strongly allergic. The allergic eczema starts to heal immediately, usually on the same day, and never erupts again. This success is achieved even if the child is not fed on a milk-free diet.

However, there are children who are not cured by this preparation. In these cases almond milk has been shown by Dr M.E. Bircher, the esteemed dietary reformer, to be a suitable substitute (see Appendix Five, p. 200). Rudolf Steiner also recommended it as a fully adequate substitute for milk. Babies only a few days old can be fed with it.

Alternatively, baby food made from soya beans (obtainable from health food shops) may help. This is also effective in treating cystitis and pyelonephritis, complaints which can be very stubborn in babies. It makes acidic urine alkaline, and can thus often treat these conditions without further medication.

9

Some General Points About Feeding Children

Diet as the child grows older

Children of a year and older gradually cut more and more teeth and therefore should do more and more chewing. They can now be given bread for breakfast and for the afternoon meal, good wholegrain bread or crispbread, never white. Good jam and honey with this should help satisfy the child's need for sweet things. If the mother cannot prevent people from giving her children sweets and chocolate, she should at least take these into her care and dole them out very sparingly. Sucking sweets must never be allowed to become a habit. It is not only the teeth that suffer. The stomach and the nervous system can also be affected because too much sugar can cause a vitamin B_1 deficiency.

Suitable savoury spreads are cream cheese or other mild soft cheeses. Sharply seasoned meat pastes and sausages are not suitable till much later, especially as most types of sausage usually contain a good deal of pork.

If after careful consideration it is decided to give the child meat, then in the early years only the white meat of young animals should be used. Broth is of no great value for children, though if slightly anaemic a child will benefit from time to time from broth made from veal bones.

It is well worth going into the matter of giving children

cereal products instead of meat. All kinds of muesli and also porridges made from various wholegrains are suitable. It is a good idea to buy these grains whole and grind them oneself just before use. The various wholegrain flakes (Demeter or Holle if possible) such as oats, barley and wheat are useful as a dish on their own when soaked in milk or juice. Highly processed and sweetened cereal products such as cornflakes or puffed wheat are not recommended.

Wholegrain foods of the kind just mentioned are also useful in encouraging lazy children to chew properly. The same can be said of almonds, hazelnuts and walnuts, which are also rich in protein and fats.

Yogurt with or without fruit is also a good food for children as are buttermilk and home-made sour milk. As regards yogurt it should be remembered, however, that it is one of the foods invented by sheep- and cattle-herding tribes whose staple diet is meat. It has been found that if eaten in large quantities by vegetarians it can upset the stomach bacteria. So care should be taken with yogurt given to small children before meat has been introduced into their diet.

When children start sharing the adults' meals, care should be taken that the food does not contain vinegar, pepper, mustard or too much salt. Salad dressings should be made with sour cream or lemon and oil. Herbs, dried or fresh, added to vegetables in small quantities are quite acceptable. Fresh herbs are even better than dried; they stimulate the digestive glands and help keep away colds of all kinds.

Children who initially object to anything new in their diet should be encouraged with words and gestures. You can introduce the meal to them as something particularly delicious! If this is unsuccessful, do not make a fuss but try again later. One should never force a child to eat. But it is also wrong to try to divert her attention with toys, radio or even television. Some children only take vegetables or even fruit if they are slightly sweetened to begin with. At about the age of five or six months sugar should be reduced and then stopped altogether.

Due to its high oxalic acid and nitrate content, artificially fertilized spinach is dangerous for babies, for these substances easily transform in the body into toxic nitrite. Biodynamic spinach is recommended instead, since it is not artificially fertilized. But never reheat this! Always throw remains away!

Some considerations when choosing food

Meat and eggs are quite superfluous for babies. Milk has plenty of protein and later curd cheese can also be added to meals several times a week. In rare cases a baby will occasionally need half an egg yolk towards the end of his first year, and this should be from a very fresh egg. Meat and broth are only necessary if the milk, cereals and other foods are of a very poor quality. If Holle and Demeter or other similar good foods are given, there need be no anxiety about the adequacy of the baby's diet.

Most potato varieties are today degenerating, so that they cannot be recommended for little children. Even as adults we feel rather dull if we have eaten too many potatoes. For children this is more far-reaching because potatoes are not good for the development of the brain. Unpolished natural rice is the best substitute for potatoes whenever possible. Millet is also good. But of course there is no harm in children eating a certain amount of potatoes, though they should never have them in the evening.

It is medically recognized that coffee, tea, alcohol and all cola drinks are highly undesirable for young children.

10

Upbringing

Early training

It has been said that we are living in the century of the child, and many parents and teachers feel that it is wrong to 'interfere with the child's freedom'. This is a complete misunderstanding of what a child needs and expects from parents and teachers alike. The very way in which she explores how far she can take naughtiness, disobedience, destructiveness and lack of respect shows that she is seeking definite guidance.

During the very early years, when she is building herself and her world through observation and imitation, she needs adults to set her an example.

Then, when she ceases to call herself by name but starts to say 'I', she begins to be aware of herself, and in order to experience herself she must of necessity come up against her surroundings. At the height of this phase she says 'no' to everything. If she is not answered with clear guidance and direction she is deeply disappointed in the depths of her being and feels driven to repeated experimental and provocative action. Through words and deeds which are in keeping with the child's comprehension, the adults around her must make it clear what is and what is not done.

With very small children rules and prohibitions of course go in one ear and out at the other. During the earlier years the child has to be shown her limits through tone of voice and consistency. Often it is more a matter of diverting her attention to something else rather than trying to establish a rule she cannot yet understand. But even an 18-month-old is quite capable of learning what is 'dirty' or 'hot', though she cannot be protected from all bad experiences. The main thing is to keep her safe from serious harm.

At the so-called 'defiant age', around three, other rules come into play. Now the child seeks conflict in order to develop her will. Every wish of the parents, however banal and ordinary, can trigger a serious dispute. The adult needs to be clear what is important enough to insist on, and what is not. It is helpful at this stage to offer the child some small scope for making her own decisions—for instance whether she wants to put on her red or blue socks (rather than debating whether she will put on socks or not), whether she would like to drink her milk from her cup or mug today, or whether she wants her teddy bear or doll to come into bed with her. In this way one can create many opportunities for the child to express her wishes and exercise her will, without entering into continual conflict. Such conflict between very unequal sides is very disadvantageous for both. If the parent continually gives in, the child eventually loses all sense of being guided, and will lose her respect for the adult. How can she imitate someone who is so much bigger and stronger than she but takes her lead from the smaller and weaker one? The adult, on the other hand, may develop a sense of resentment towards the child because she feels tyrannized.

If, on the other hand, the child is always subordinate, she will soon feel misunderstood and unloved, and her interest in the world and her own ego will soon diminish, as will her courage to make new discoveries.

Thus sensible parents will formulate their commands in a way that can be implemented without great compulsion. For instance, it is relatively easy to get a child to sit quietly at mealtimes, but forcing her to eat against her will is well-nigh impossible. It is the same with sleeping: one can demand that a child goes to her room at bedtime, but sleep itself cannot be commanded.

Of course one must have self-discipline. At table, particularly, many bad habits can be passed on. It will be difficult to get a child to eat peacefully if adults themselves are continually jumping up and running about.

By making 'mischief' a child is often just trying to draw attention to herself, and instead of a telling off may just need more loving interest.

It is most important in bringing up children to avoid being uncertain and anxious. This is simply annoying for a healthy child and is in itself a temptation to defiance, whereas for a sick child it is a burden that disturbs and even prevents her from getting well.

The child's urge to be active

There are divergent opinions about the degree to which children should be restricted during their early years. In western countries the tendency is to leave them almost entirely free. The consequence of this can be increasingly wild behaviour by children who almost terrorize their families, visitors and even neighbours till finally the exasperated parents see nothing for it but to dump them in front of the television screen to keep them quiet—which in fact only exacerbates the problem, as television has been found to induce hyperactivity in many children.

Children are left excessively free out of a kind of sentimental misunderstanding of what a child needs from those who bring her up. In fact neither unlimited freedom to fidget and rush about nor too much restriction is good for the child. As with everything, the happy medium has to be found. For considerations regarding the balance between firm wrapping and letting the small baby kick, see pages 79–80.

As the child continues to grow, the proper use of the playpen or walker will be the next question to crop up. This useful apparatus can be damaging if seen simply as a means of curbing the fidgetiness of an active child or if it is used to imprison a child who is too wild. But with proper use it gives the baby for a few hours each day a little realm of her own, while freeing others from having to keep a watchful eye on her every minute of her waking hours. Efforts have been made by some manufacturers to make less cagelike playpens.

Rocking is another important element in upbringing. A baby rocked in a cradle for her first few months is most unlikely to grow into a child who later develops the habit of sitting up in bed in the evening or even in the middle of the night rocking to and fro to the accompaniment of her own rhythmical sing-song. Later, nothing could be better than a hammock, rocking chair or rocking horse to satisfy her fundamental need for rhythmical movement. In contrast, the bouncing chairs and seats now available on the market go against the natural swinging rhythm of breathing. The child's obvious enjoyment of this bouncing movement is not necessarily the only criterion, for she will delight in any kind of motion and activity.

So, give the child freedom to move about and be active within normal limits, and she will not need periods of excessively wild romping and rushing that do her no good. There will be a period when nothing will be safe from the baby and she will need constant supervision, but this is unavoidable. Later she will continue to satisfy her need to move by climbing about on the apparatuses in children's playgrounds, and with her scooter, tricycle, or toboggan in winter. When she is five or six she can begin to learn to swim.

Play

For children, play is pure artistry and serves no practical purpose. When they are undisturbed by adults they play with dreamy and dedicated absorption. Indeed, a small child who places her building bricks exactly and neatly one upon the other is not playing, but is entering prematurely into an intellectual element. It is not good to disturb a child who is absorbed in a game of her own, specially not to give her adult advice about how her play should proceed. On the other hand, if she wants to tell you about her games, listen seriously and do not criticize or make too many suggestions. A child's games are like beautiful dreams and their influence will remain with her all her life.

The capacities for concentration and active, creative engagement with one's environment which play develops is a vital preparation for later learning at school, and indeed for all of life.

Toys should be of natural, healthy materials (wood, wool or silk, natural dyes). Strident colours, plastic materials and toys that make electrical noises harm the development of the child's senses. In infancy the child is learning about the world through all her senses, drinking it in as it were, and natural materials give her an intuitive sense of the world as a true, solid and sustaining place.

Do not be surprised or upset when the oldest and shabbiest teddy is more beloved than the beautiful new doll. Try to arrange with grandparents and godparents that presents should be given so that the child is not submerged in toys. And if she has too many, hide some for a while and let them appear again later on.

Up to the age of about six, children do not clearly distinguish between imagination and reality. Ideally this phase can last even longer. At this age fairy tales also have their rightful and powerful place; through them the child learns to know the world, to meet such qualities as love, hate, faithfulness and trickery embodied in the figures and characters who people these stories.

Free painting on white paper with watercolours (not filling in pre-drawn pictures!) is a most satisfying artistic play activity, as is modelling with coloured wax.

It is best to wait at least till she starts school before giving the child mechanical toys, and it is to be hoped that fathers who long for electric trains will wait till their boys are about ten years old.

Far more damage than is realized is done by allowing children to embark too early on a new phase.

So-called bad habits

A number of so-called 'bad habits' in children are nothing more than imitation or a game and should not be judged from a moral standpoint. 'Thefts' of money or trinkets, nibbling food or sweets on the sly, taking toys and other objects to pieces are all things that can be dealt with by understanding parents and teachers. Even tormenting or killing insects and worms is probably no more than a misplaced desire to explore the world. Parents and teachers could do well to seek the origin of the 'bad habit' in their own behaviour. Certainly they should try to think *with* the child rather than against her in order to get to the bottom of what might be causing the problem. Once they have found the cause, gentle guidance and understanding will usually be sufficient to bring it to an end.

Similarly when little children play with their genitals it is nonsense to talk of masturbation. A bored child left sitting on the potty for too long is quite likely to fiddle about, but there is no more to this than if she were to pick her nose or bite her nails. If the parents react with horror and indignation, however, the child will start to have all sorts of suspicions. So instead of smacking or scolding, simply give her something else to do with her hands. Also avoid leaving her on the potty for too long in the first place and see that she does not lie awake for hours in bed. Inflammation of the genitals arising from a chill or the rubbing of tight clothes can also turn the child's attention too much in that direction.

The facts of life

Up to as late as the tenth year a child's questions about her origin are concerned fundamentally with her spiritual origins. The facts of physical conception and birth only become really comprehensible when the ability to observe objectively and think abstractly starts to develop. Thus early explanations and, worse still, practical demonstrations completely miss the point and show a total misunderstanding of the child's being and development.

The small child is non-sexual. Interest and understanding for sexual processes starts to emerge with the onset of puberty between the ages of 12 and 15 years. Parallel with it the young person's own moral capacities and thought life begin to awaken. Till then she lives more within the feelings and ideas of those around her. Thus the examples set by uninhibited sensuality or sensible and serious behaviour will have definite effects on the way she enters and copes with puberty and her awakening sexual urges.

Other aspects that affect the onset of puberty lie much earlier on in the child's life. Overfeeding, especially with eggs and meat, causes infants to lose their childlike qualities and grow up too quickly, and later on puberty is likely to be early and difficult. For the same reason pepper, paprika, mustard and vinegar, and even too much salt, are unsuitable in the diet of small children. Overstimulation of the senses, e.g. constant background noise from radio and television, glaring and overbright decor in the child's surroundings accompanied by too many toys, too many different new foods and tastes all at once, cause children to mature physically more quickly than they should, which in turn means that puberty arrives before the child's mental and emotional development can cope with it.

Bed wetting

By the age of two-and-a-half the child should be clean and dry by day and night. A proper relationship between waking and sleeping is established, and this in turn determines the excretory functions. Constant wetting by day and night can have many causes. The child may have a bladder complaint, or simply a chill caused by insufficient warm clothing for the lower half of her body. Or there may be a psychological problem such as jealousy of siblings, definite fears, environmental disturbances, etc. In most cases the doctor will be able to assist either with medicaments (Weleda) or with advice. When the bed wetting stops, there will also be positive effects on the child's soul life and development.

If a child still wets the bed at the age of four, then it is time to do something about it to avoid emotional or physical repercussions.

Blame and reproach is of no use at all. Such children may simply be having difficulty in leaving an earlier stage behind. They may not yet have fully established the connection with their own body, right into the lower body and the tips of the toes. Check whether the bed is comfortable and warm. Are the potty or toilet easy to reach and appealing to use?

If a child has cold feet in the evening, first check shoes and socks are warm, then give her a warming footbath several evenings in a row (see section on water treatments, page 185).

If she is sleeping restlessly, give her a yarrow compress

placed on the stomach, wrapped in a towel around the body with a light hot water bottle on top, all firmly wrapped in a broad woollen cloth and fixed in place with safety pins. Take this off carefully after 1 to 3 hours, without waking the child.

For general 'irritability' give her a bladder-calming remedy, such as Cantharis 4x, 5 drops daily.

If these measures do not help it is best to consult a doctor to ensure there is no organic disorder of the kidneys or bladder.

One remedy that has proved helpful is to massage copper ointment 0.4% into the stomach above the bladder. You can also give Vesica urinalis 4x or Hypericum 4x, 5 drops three times daily.

If bed wetting continues into primary school age this requires much patience but always stops eventually. In older children an artistic therapy is helpful, particularly eurythmy therapy but also music therapy.

Punishment, moral pressure or even rewards should never be used, as this can drive the problem into another sphere where it may become unreachable.

Thumb sucking

The same applies to thumb sucking or nail biting. A newborn child immediately begins to suck if her mouth comes into contact with anything. With increasing age this natural reflex is replaced by chewing as the child is gradually given solid food. She can now sit at table and start to eat and drink independently, in imitation of the others. The mother needs to lovingly support this move towards more independence and not feed her too long through worry about messes—but nor should she let the child play around at will during eating. There will be a transition phase where the child may still be sucking on the bottle as well as eating solids, but one should try to avoid continual sucking all day long. There may be a particular situation when it is called for. Likewise one can carefully observe how the child uses a much-beloved 'pinky' or sucking cloth: is the child using it to create a little pause in activity, and afterwards returning to play with fresh gusto? Or is it more a sign of taking flight and refuge from a situation the child is not coping with? Or a sign or apathy or boredom?

If we see that the child is sucking in a relaxed, happy way, either on a bottle or her thumb, then that is fine. But if her breathing is shallow and quick, her eyes glassy, and if she sucks in a way that seems turned in on herself, that is a habit to discourage.

The mother should observe the child carefully and see if she lacks something. Does she need more peace and quiet, more attention or more stimulation? Can the mother perhaps give the child a bit more sense of protection at night when she says goodnight, maybe with a special verse or song, which gives her more courage for the next day?

One should focus attention particularly on the period after the age of three, when children start wanting to take an active part in the life of adults and to imitate everything. If one does not suppress this urge to activity and to become independent, but calmly allows the child to join in with a purposeful, peaceful activity of some kind, for instance helping with sweeping or cleaning, then the substitute, passive activity of sucking will become superfluous.

The infant's sleep

The alternation between sleeping and waking is very strongly linked to the rhythm of breathing. The day's experiences are expressed in the breathing, and thus sleep is affected via the breath. This effect manifests right into the child's dreams, possibly giving rise to frightening dreams, oppressive feelings and even stomach cramps. In healthy sleeping periods the upbuilding, renewing forces become active, while too little sleep promotes susceptibility to illness.

The day-night rhythm is only gradually established. Children aged one to two still need a few hours' sleep in the morning and evening. And until the child reaches school age a midday sleep is healthy and usually also necessary. A midday rest is important at this age, even if the child does not sleep. When the child reaches school age, twelve hours of sleep a night are still necessary.

In general children nowadays sleep too little. This is caused by lack of rhythm in the adult world, the many distractions and noises, and parents' lack of awareness of the importance of sufficient sleep.

If, during the day, one considers the infant's capacities and does not continually give her new, unknown experiences to deal with, but allows her to discover her environment in a way appropriate to her age, then her breathing will also grow regular. She will be happy to go to bed, and will fall asleep easily, her arms upwards.

Those who learn to sleep properly in childhood will not need sleeping pills when they grow up.

Fear and anxiety

Most of us will remember the fears suffered during child-hood, the fear of dogs and other animals, caterwauling in the garden at night that we took for the crying of children, creaking noises in furniture and floors, or even fear of certain people.

Fear is often occasioned by noises that are not understood or by the first inklings of animal urges and instincts. Often children also tune in to the existential fear that afflicts so many adults these days.

Strangely enough, the fears experienced by children during bombing raids in the last war appear to have left no noticeable psychological scars. But it seems that the shocks had a direct influence on the life forces themselves, for many people have subsequently come to suffer physically from a marked constitutional weakness. Fear disturbs the building-up processes and cramps the blood vessels.

Often the doctor only hears about a child's fears by chance during consultations about 'proper' illnesses. This is partly because parents know from experience that they are likely to be given nothing more than a sedative, which they instinctively feel will not do the child any good. Or they may be under the impression that psychological problems cannot be helped with medicines. Thus many children suffer agonies for years when they could quite well be helped by the doctor.

Unfortunately many parents still bring up their children with the help of hints about the 'bogeyman' or some other threatening character. Fears can also arise as a result of television or radio programmes, or even a visit to a circus or the zoo. Children cannot absorb too many impressions, especially those which are incomprehensible to them. These undigested experiences then reappear in their dreams. Even an evening meal that is too heavy can cause nightly fears. If a child has a nightmare, make sure that she wakes up fully, if necessary by wiping her face with a cold sponge. She will then usually go to sleep again quite peacefully after a comforting chat. If there is anything that frightens her, remove it if possible. Often a dim lamp in the bedroom does wonders.

But if the child is not comforted by ordinary means, a doctor should definitely be consulted. Sometimes childhood fears can lead to neuroses later.

Radio and television

Some people feel that even small babies need constant background music from the radio. Later they allow their children to do their homework while the radio is on. Some children are so addicted that they imagine they cannot even do their homework unless the radio is blaring. And the television has encroached even further on social and family life, to the extent that it often determines daily routine.

Daily doses of television work on the child in the following way: a profusion of scenes that cannot possibly be assimilated psychologically pass before her eyes in rapid succession. School work begins to suffer, not necessarily because the children are distracted from finishing their homework and go to bed too late, but because the agitating rapid sequence of pictures causes a high degree of physical fidgetiness. Moreover, soul activity and creativity of will remain underdeveloped.

It is now known that television can cause a number of serious medical conditions: damage to eyes and ears; heart and circulatory disturbances (TV angina pectoris); and above all postural damage (TV neck). Latent epilepsy can also be activated. A number of hospitals now have special departments in their paediatric clinics for TV-damaged children.

If a child's tummy is upset through the consumption of food that disagrees with her, steps are taken to make sure that she does not eat the same dish again. Yet if a child's constitution is spoilt by radio and television this is not even noticed, mainly because people are not aware that this is a possibility. The disturbance and damage may not be very noticeable, but it is serious because the child's physical organs are still being completed as she grows, and their ultimate delicacy or grossness is largely dependent on the sense impressions to which she is subject during this process.

Pre-school learning—a disaster

For a number of years now pre-school learning has been described as representing a decisive advantage by educationalists intent on being progressive. They say that children both can and want to start learning much earlier, that their ability to learn is particularly great during the first four years and that by the fourth year 50% of their intelligence is either developed or lost for ever. They hold that talent is not something with which children are born but that they can be educated to have it and that as the social environment is more important than heredity one must start early to promote intellectual capacity by giving the children stimulating tasks.

None of these statements is absolutely wrong and they are

a good example of how half-truths are often more dangerous and difficult to shift than outright errors or lies. They are based on the view that the faculties of children three to five years old are being wasted and that they are insufficiently educated if they have not been taught to read from the age of three.

Reform efforts of this kind, however, must be based on very fundamental knowledge of the child's nature. The demands sound so obvious and seem quite logical but they completely disregard the real laws of child development.

We have all met examples of these precocious and prematurely old children and seen the way their ambitious parents show off their party tricks. In extreme cases they are infant prodigies who develop really spectacular achievements at a very early age. But follow them into later life and you will find that the overwhelming majority become pitiful creatures whose creative forces have all been exhausted in childhood. At best they become completely one-sided specialists in some narrow field, not complete human beings able to think, feel and act harmoniously.

All parents can observe how a small baby cries with might and main, becoming bright red and really showing her fury. This strengthens her breathing. A little later they see how she practises tirelessly with her little hands, watching them as they move. Then she starts to kick, to pull herself up and to crawl. And finally she learns to walk and run about, falling often, picking herself up and running on, beaming with delight. She grows steadier, arms and legs come under control and her balance improves. She really works at becoming oriented in space. Soon her activities extend to her scooter and her tricycle, and her arms are also used increasingly as she 'helps' her

mother with housework and copies every activity she sees
around her. She tirelessly exercises her speech organs and the
muscles which help her see and touch. In short, for the first
seven years the child has an untameable primeval urge to be
active in every possible way with her body.

Now it is essential to recognize that all this activity of limbs
and all movable parts of the body including every muscle of
the metabolic organs has one common denominator: the
development of the will. All these activities are subject to the
will, partly consciously and partly unconsciously. The
stimulus for all movements, except reflex actions, comes from
the will forces of the soul which in a way grasp the limbs from
the outside and lead them to whatever the soul feels as a wish.
Only muscles can actually move. The inner process of every
movement is made possible by complicated metabolic processes which remain in the unconscious unless there are
injuries or illnesses such as rheumatism. All kinds of movement are expressions of will.

So far we have described only the external aspect of
movement. There is also an internal aspect which leads us
into the most intimate part of human nature. Where are we
most ourselves? In thoughts and words we can dissemble or
lie and give out knowledge we have read in books as our own
creation. It is in our actions that we reveal our most intimate
intentions. Our acts of will reveal our personality and in the
final analysis determine our destiny. Even consciously linking
one thought to another is only possible through the will.

This is the depth and breadth required for understanding
the development of the will life. And to develop all the
possibilities of her will a child needs the first seven years of her
life from birth until she changes her teeth. Every minute is

filled to bursting with this process and not an instant is lost. Through ceaseless movement in the first seven years the will is developed.

However, this development can be disregarded and brought into disharmony. We can do gymnastics with a one-year-old or teach her to swim. Though this is too early for regimented movement, at least it is movement. But if we cause the child to use her intellectual capacities in reading and writing while she is still too young and should be developing her will through movement, we make her use up forces which are not yet mature and which later in life will be sorely lacking as a result. That many children enter happily into this kind of activity is no justification, for all children enjoy being at the centre of adult attention. It is also no excuse to say that we are not forcing children but are leading them to reading and writing through play. Childish play should be entirely undirected externally and involve only the imagination and the will but not the intellect.

It will be the doctors who find themselves dealing with the consequences of pre-school learning. The surplus vitality needed by adults to cope with life and work in the world are used up in childhood so that the very opposite happens to the ideal imagined by the advocates of pre-school learning: ability and efficiency decrease instead of increasing. The beginning of this can be seen in the children themselves when they grow pale, sleep badly, grow slowly and tire easily. Conversely the results of a childhood without early learning and with plenty of time to develop the will properly can be seen in some of the grand old men of our time such as Churchill, Adenauer, Henry Ford or Nelson Mandela who all had childhood days without the problems of early intellectual training.

One of the greatest fallacies of today is the belief that whatever is possible is also permissible; innumerable things are possible, but to do many of them is utter foolishness or worse.

So far as the development of the will is concerned, what a child needs until the change of teeth is not pre-school training but a good kindergarten where her will forces can be developed in a meaningful way. Her learning at this age is not intellectual but mainly imaginative play and physical action based on imitation.

11

The Sick Child

1. GENERAL POINTS

What is illness?

Why should man, the pinnacle of creation, suffer from so many illnesses? If he were the same as any natural creation, stone, plant, animal, there would be no inner reasons for him to become ill. But because of his spiritual aspect, man rises above nature, he is a citizen of both the natural and the spiritual world. He has developed beyond his links with nature and now lives in a conflict between the natural and the spiritual part of his total being.

With his physical body and the etheric life forces working in it, he is more or less subject to the laws of the natural world. But with his soul and spirit he has separated himself from the life of nature. This inner contrast is the source of his special human capabilities and achievements, but it also contains the possibility of aberrations and mistakes, and of disturbances of inner harmony that are the cause of all illnesses. Man has achieved the ability to live and act in opposition to ancient, divine spiritual laws; he is on the way to achieving freedom of action, but he has to pay for this with the possibility of disease. Having lost his instinct for what is good and right, he has opened the door to sin, disease and death.

How does healing take place?

It is the anthroposophical doctor's task to stimulate and strengthen the patient's life forces so that the body can heal itself. This is indeed the aim of all healing and of the medicines used.

There is a fundamental distinction, however, between the method of doctors who use medicines derived from nature and those who use synthetic medicines. A chemical medicine contains no living forces and it can therefore not stimulate a healing process, since dead materials cannot bring about living processes. A chemical medicine can, though, have chemical effects, for instance the dulling of pain or the killing of bacteria, but there is an accompanying danger of damage to living forces. The anthroposophical and homoeopathic doctor uses preparations derived from natural animal, plant and mineral substances, and with these he is able to affect not only the physical body but also the life forces working in it. It is his aim to strengthen these forces so that they can themselves take on the healing of the illness.

The healing power of fever

The ego, the spiritual centre of the personality, has already been mentioned a number of times as the force which welds together the other three members of man into a totality. The ego is the 'master of the house', keeping order and seeking to keep out intruders. But if something foreign, for instance poison, cold or bacteria, does manage to enter, the ego has to do battle. Its weapon is an increase in body temperature, in other words a fever. A fever brings about reactions and calls all life forces to the defence. The doctor can work with a fever and there are even means of bringing on a beneficial fever. The intruding foreign influence is 'digested' more thoroughly than food by means of the fever.

Thus the ego's efforts can be supported by the use of hot compresses, sweat treatment and baths, and preparations that raise the body temperature. In the last resort, all efforts to restore order in the body's 'household' stem from the ego, with the resulting symptoms in the organism of the life forces. Thus so long as inflammation and temperature correspond with one another, there is no danger.

Fever is an integral part of many illnesses. Often a critical situation arises if there is no fever, or if it has been suppressed. There is no cause for concern when the state of the illness and the degree of temperature correspond with each other. I have twice met with children who were perfectly well three days after having had a temperature of 107.7°F (42.3°C).

Keeping warm in bed

The fever processes instigated by the ego require calm and protection provided by the layers of bedding. One should ensure proper covering and blankets. The child should neither get too cold nor too hot. Resting in bed is also necessary to prevent the forces needed for recovery from being dissipated, as happens through over-cooling, restless activity and excessive sensory impressions. A quiet environment, gentle light, a well-aired room promote the healing process. Complications and relapses are often a result of not observing this basic rule.

It is often difficult to keep infants in bed, especially when they are only slightly ill. Nevertheless it is worth persevering, or at least to enclose the child in warmth and peace in the home environment, to quieten the business of a normal day and spend the days of illness quietly and intimately with the child. These quiet times will continue to work as sources of strength right in to old age, and are the focus of many childhood memories.

It is a good idea to have some special 'illness games' which the child can play when sick, perhaps also on his own, which are put away again once the child recovers.

2. ACUTE ILLNESSES

Birth damage

A newborn baby can have considerable swellings on his head resulting from the birth process. These are filled with liquid and can be quite large. They should be examined immediately, but are nearly always harmless and disappear rapidly, especially after the application of Mercurialis ointment (Weleda). Sometimes considerable growths remain, which disappear more slowly. Some swellings on the head are more serious, however.

On the other hand, the distortions of the skull that can come about during birth are nearly always quite harmless and disappear within a few days. Fortunately the individual bones of the skull are not yet firmly anchored and so can yield to the pressure. Parents therefore do not need to be alarmed if their baby's head displays a decidedly startling shape when they first see him. This will soon rectify itself.

If during the early weeks the baby is obviously clumsy

about taking the breast or cannot seem to learn to take a proper hold, or if he is excessively passive, the doctor should be informed. There may be a brain haemorrhage, which is fairly frequent though rarely with lasting ill effects. If it is serious, the consequences are unconsciousness, cramps or unwillingness to drink.

The doctor should also be called if the baby's skin begins to turn yellow during the first day. 'Normal' jaundice of the newborn does not set in till the second or third day and usually disappears after two or three weeks. Premature babies retain the yellowish colouring longer, as do congenitally retarded children.

Not infrequently the baby's collar bone is broken during birth. Usually this mends by itself without treatment, but the doctor must decide whether anything should be done.

Ailments during the early months

There can be a swelling of the breast glands in both boys and girls soon after birth as a result of hormonal adjustment. This contains so-called 'lac neonatorum', which should not be expelled from the breast by squeezing. It is much better to leave the swelling alone or apply Mercurialis ointment and it will disappear quite soon.

Bleeding from the navel after the remainder of the umbilical cord has been discarded can also cause mothers anxiety, but this is quite harmless so long as the navel has been kept scrupulously clean. The bleeding can be stopped quite easily, for instance by applying an arnica dressing (10 drops Weleda Arnica 20% in half a cup of water). The doctor will only have to be called in rare cases.

Wild flesh sometimes grows in the navel making a lump as big as a cherry stone or even a hazel nut. In this case too, the doctor must be consulted. It is essential to keep the navel absolutely clean until the wound is quite healed. If despite these precautions there should be signs of swelling, redness or dampness, or a bad smell or pus, or a hernia or growth, the doctor must be consulted. Regarding umbilical and other hernias see the next section.

Newborn babies quite often have pink birthmarks of different sizes, usually symmetrically situated on both halves of the head, particularly on the forehead, the eyelids, the nose, the back of the head and the back of the neck. These are caused by an enlargement of blood vessels and usually disappear before the child is 15 months old, though in the nape of the neck they sometimes remain longer. They are quite harmless and require no treatment.

Another kind of birthmark is more serious. These, too, are caused by an enlargement of blood vessels but they are thicker and resemble dark red sponges which empty when pressed and then fill again with blood. These are not present at birth but grow during the early months, sometimes at considerable speed. Rapid growths of this kind can be dangerous and should be under constant observation. Recent research in America has shown that the rapid growth of these birthmarks usually ceases at about the tenth month, though in some cases it continues till the child is two or more. Then they gradually disappear by themselves leaving only a hardly noticeable colouration of the skin by the time the child is six. This happens even if the birthmarks are large and thick. So parents should not urge the doctor to treat these marks, for no known methods have such good cosmetic results as self-healing. On the contrary, they lead to more or less permanent scarring. Since these marks are often on the face or other visible parts it takes courage to wait, but it is worth it.

Other birthmarks, brown or black moles with or without hairs, are said to be the result of the mother receiving a shock during pregnancy. If this were so, what would babies have looked like born to mothers who went through the horrors of the blitz while pregnant!

The neck muscles are sometimes damaged during birth, and the baby will then bend his head towards the painful side. Usually this will heal on its own, but occasionally the baby's head remains bent to one side. Usually this can be remedied with massage and applications of Mercurialis ointment, but just occasionally a small operation is necessary.

If forceps are used during the birth, this sometimes damages some of the facial muscles. The baby's mouth will then be crooked when he cries, or perhaps one eyelid will not close properly. The arm nerves can also be damaged, but this nearly always heals of its own accord.

Phimosis is quite common in infant boys. This is a narrowing of the foreskin which can cause difficulty in passing water. Usually the doctor can correct this during the early weeks by stretching. The foreskin finally stretches by itself during puberty.

In baby girls there is sometimes bleeding or a sticky discharge from the vagina. Like the breast swelling this is probably hormonal in origin and it is quite harmless, ceasing after a few days.

Hernias

The most common of these is the umbilical hernia. The naval sometimes does not heal properly when the remains of the umbilical cord have fallen away. A round, usually hard, lump is felt under the skin and can be easily pressed back into the tummy. However, when the baby cries or presses when passing a motion it is liable to pop out again and the hole tends to stretch, so that the lump can reach the size of a walnut or even more.

Above and below the navel, hernias of the abdominal wall can also occur. In the embryo, the abdominal wall grows together from both sides, but sometimes it does not knit together sufficiently in the middle, so that a slit is left open. A portion of the intestines can become pinched in this, which is very painful.

In less serious cases only the external skin bulges. Gentle pressure pushes the air back into the abdomen and the bulge disappears.

In both cases the doctor will apply a sticking plaster to hold the place closed in a fold of skin. This enables the weak part to shrink and grow together. Take care to dry the plaster well after bathing, as it should remain for some time. If necessary replace it with a fresh one. The small baby may need the plaster for three to four months. But if the hernia occurs later than eight or nine months the plaster method is no longer effective. The child will then need a small operation later.

On the whole, umbilical hernias are not dangerous, although especially with girls they must be properly healed in view of the strain placed on the wall of the abdomen in pregnancy later on. Inguinal hernias (in the groin) can be much more serious, especially in boys, where intestines can be pushed right down into the scrotum, leading sometimes to strangulation of the intestine.

When a child cries with pain and cannot be soothed it is possible that the cause may be a hernia of this kind. Examine the groin on both sides. There will be a hard lump painful to the touch and the baby will cry continuously and keep stretching his legs. Place the baby in a warm bath or apply damp warm compresses to the swelling. If this does not cause the hernia to retract, the doctor must be called immediately, even in the middle of the night. The strangulation must not be allowed to continue for more than six hours. The doctor will probably be able to press the protruding part back into the abdomen, which immediately removes the pain as well as the danger. If he is unsuccessful the child will have to have a swift operation. But quite often the bumping of the car on the way to the hospital causes the hernia to slip back.

Even tiny babies can be operated on if the hernia is acute, but it is better to wait till the child is more than a year old, using a rubber truss till then. In very thin children the hernia can close as a result of a rapid increase in weight, which can be achieved with a change of diet. Hernias in the groin are far more frequent in boys than in girls.

Rickets—history and incidence

Rickets occurs when there is insufficient assimilation of sunlight resulting in insufficient transformation of the pro-vitamin in the skin into vitamin D. In consequence the organism fails to absorb sufficient mineral salts, especially calcium, from the food eaten. The bones and connective tissues remain soft and watery, there is bending of some bones and enlargement at the ends of others, for instance the knobbed appearance of the ribs where they join the cartilage of the breastbone. The bones at the back of the skull can become soft and flattened. And lack of tissue firmness in lungs and other internal organs weakens their functioning and gives rise to the tendency for catarrhal complaints, diarrhoea and other conditions. Directly connected with this delay in mineralization of the body is a slowness of soul development: grasping, sitting, standing, speaking, and thinking are not achieved at the normal rate.

As a whole the disease can be characterized as a retardation of the incarnation of the formative forces of the soul and spirit, or as a retention of embryonic forms and qualities.

In the mid-twenties of the last century Professor Windaus developed artificial vitamin D and this led to a fundamental change in the rickets situation as it existed then. In some countries a prophylactic treatment was developed consisting of a few massive doses of vitamin D administered to babies during the early weeks of life. The effect was a spectacular hardening of the bones and connective tissues and it seemed as if the rickets problem was solved for good. Anyone trying to point out the disadvantages of this treatment was shouted down.

My own negative attitude to it began in the very early days of its application when I conducted an autopsy on a baby. I found that it had died from arteriosclerosis, a disease of old age.

In the months during which I was engaged with this case my medical thinking was influenced in a particular way. I came to the following conclusion: Human life flows like a river which is bound by certain laws and certain periodic developments during which specific advances take place. The baby learns to grasp, to sit, to stand, to speak, to think and so on. Then comes the middle period of life, and finally old age with its characteristic symptoms. Here, however, was a baby who had died from a disease of advancing age. I realized that the speed of life's stream can be altered and that it is not necessarily bound to rigid laws.

As time went on it became more and more apparent that large and even small doses of vitamin D were leading to the permanent illness or death of children. An extensive literature is now available on the subject and in most countries the treatment has been discontinued in favour of a much longer treatment with very small doses.

There are, however, still some who favour the massive dose treatment, saying that mothers are too neglectful and will not persist in administering small doses over a long period. This may be true in a few cases, but to most mothers it is an insult. And even if a few are negligent, this is no reason for continuing such a dangerous treatment across the board.

The symptoms of vitamin D poisoning are initially constipation, followed by persistent lack of appetite and slowing down of development, vomiting, headache, hardening of the bones, kidney failure. The symptoms are usually at their worst 30 to 60 days after the dose has been administered.

In my opinion there is yet another aspect to be considered in this matter. The too rapid and too concentrated mineralization of the child's body brought about by massive dose treatment is accompanied by a speeding up of the rest of the child's development. Just as the body grows old too soon, so consciousness awakes too rapidly. To the misguided joy of some parents the children are precociously forward by the time they go to school. Many, however, begin to fall behind by the time they are ten or twelve. Though physically robust and often astonishingly tall, they fail in intellectual ability and teachers complain of lack of concentration, inattentiveness, nervous fidgetiness and lack of interest. Consciousness becomes narrowed down to a few specialized subjects and there is difficulty in thinking. There are, of course, also other factors which speed up the development of children today, in particular the ever-growing influence of technology all around us.

In recent years the rickets cases seen by doctors have not only once again increased in number but have also become more serious than they have been for a long time and are sometimes combined with symptoms of tetany. The reasons for the increase and the accompanying symptoms are not exactly known, but it is my conviction that a decisive role is played by the increase in the amount of unsuitable foods given to babies: dried milk products, farinaceous products with no nutritional value, and tinned vegetables. Fortunately the disease is never as extreme now as it used to be.

Every newborn baby, even if breastfed, is in danger of contracting rickets. Some are particularly susceptible, for instance babies whose mothers are particularly anaemic or suffer from calcium deficiency, babies born during the dark winter months, and also premature or weak babies. There are also families with an inherited tendency for rickets. Overfed babies and those fed mainly on dried milk products are also more in danger. Furthermore, the haze of pollution over industrial towns has now reached a stage where on many days the sun's ultraviolet rays can hardly penetrate through to the earth.

Rickets—prevention and treatment

So many requests have reached me from worried parents all over the world who know the dangers of vitamin D that I have decided to give in detail my method of preventing and treating rickets based on anthroposophical medicine. But parents should if possible consult their own doctor first. Perhaps he could read this section and then adjust the treatment to the individual case. They should also take the child to see him about once a month while the treatment lasts.

As has been said, rickets is becoming more frequent and virtually every child could contract the disease. Therefore prevention should start as early as five or six weeks. This applies particularly when the parents themselves have suffered from rickets, but also if the child is born in the winter months when there is little daylight or if the family lives in rather dark accommodation.

It must be stated categorically that treatment with calcium alone, even with the otherwise excellent Weleda Calcium Supplements I and II, is not a sufficiently dependable preventive method.

Even breastfed babies can contract rickets, though the danger is far smaller than with bottle-fed infants. For the latter the advice on nutrition given in this book, particularly concerning the use of Demeter and Holle products, is especially important for the prevention of rickets. Over-feeding increases the probability of the disease.

It is important to remember that the illness is caused by lack of sunlight. Phosphorous can increase the effects of the available sunlight or act as a substitute when it is lacking. This is given in a homoeopathic potency, usually 6x. Starting at about the fifth week, give the baby three drops morning and midday in a little water. Continue for four to six weeks and then pause for a week or a fortnight. In addition to this it is important to give in the morning a small saltspoon of calcium phosphate (apatite 6x or calcium phosphoricum 6x) and in the evening a saltspoon of calcium carbonate (conchae verae 10x or calcium carbonicum 10x). All these are given before meals in a little water.

In special cases cod liver oil continues to prove useful. Choose a brand which is pure and natural and give the child one teaspoon twice daily if it does not upset his digestion.

In the case of rickety children whose parents have also suffered from the disease it is essential that they be taken to the doctor, if possible one who works with natural treatments. In those who have inherited the illness even massive dose treatment with vitamin D has been known to fail. It is a matter of treating the whole constitution of the child.

A final cure of rickets takes time to achieve. Parents must therefore be patient, for it is not only a matter of a lack of solidity in the bones but also one of a disturbance in the process of incarnation. This tendency to develop too slowly must be overcome gently and not by force. In recent years it has frequently been stated in the relevant literature that a mild affliction of rickets need not be feared nearly as much as the danger of kidney, brain or heart disease caused by synthetic vitamin D. Certainly the opposite of rickets, an artificial speeding up of the development and excessive hardening of the bones together with a tendency to arteriosclerosis, is a threat to health and strength which will follow a person throughout life. Conversely, rickets, except in serious or neglected cases, can be overcome during childhood with suitable treatment and then very rarely leaves a residue of bone deformation.

Apart from the above treatment with medicine, which it is up to the mother to carry out carefully and punctually, there are further possibilities for maintaining the child's health. The child's food must be of the best possible quality and contain enough natural vitamins and above all plenty of minerals. The Demeter and Holle products described in this book have proved excellent as aids to rickets prevention. It is essential for the baby to have gruels and puddings made with cereals and later to eat wholegrain bread. A child with a large fontanel and other indications of rickets will need root vegetables and their raw juices, particularly carrots, from about the fourth month.

Another aid in preventing rickets is plenty of fresh air and sunlight or outdoor daylight if the sun is not shining. In winter if it is windy and rather cold it is sufficient to take the child out for half or quarter of an hour. If a balcony or garden is available the child can be left out in his pram for hours if he is well wrapped up and tucked in with a hot water bottle. Strong east winds are dangerous however.

In the summer the child can be out of doors much longer and when this is not possible his cot should be placed directly beside the open window. On hot days he can be placed naked in the sun for a short while, first about two minutes on his back and two on his tummy. This can be gradually increased to about 15 minutes. It is pointless to aim for a sun tan as quickly as possible because brown skin keeps the sun's rays out. Also it is important to remember that as a general rule the head, that is the brain and the spinal fluid, must not have too much sun, if only because this can promote the development of polio.

The value of a canopy of light red material (see page 65) has already been mentioned. This protects the baby from the inflammatory rays of the sun while letting through those which help prevent rickets. So under such a canopy the baby can be given much more sunlight than would be possible without.

Finally there are bath mixtures which help combat rickets. Those containing thyme are specially useful. Sulphur bath mixtures (Weleda or others) can also be used if available. These are given three times per week in courses of 12 baths.

Diarrhoea

Diarrhoea is rare in breastfed babies and is usually a symptom of trouble in some other organ. In bottle-fed babies, diarrhoea and other intestinal disorders are more frequent.

During the first three months in particular it must be taken quite seriously and treated immediately. The danger of the complaint is that it causes rapid dehydration and loss of mineral salts. Dietary mistakes, but also overheating caused by too much bedding, specially during the summer, can cause diarrhoea.

The first measure is to cease giving milk, fat and sugar (this applies to diarrhoea in children of all ages). Small amounts of camomile tea or very weak ordinary tea are given, if necessary with a tiny amount of sweetener. During the first three months of life, babies must not be deprived of milk for more than two or three days, so if this is necessary the doctor will prescribe a suitable alternative diet. A useful remedial recipe is carrot soup: boil a pound of fresh carrots for at least two hours in a litre of water with a large pinch of salt. Strain, saving the water and topping up to bring back to one litre. Pass the carrots twice through a fine sieve, then return the pulp to the water. Feed the baby with this mixture for five or more meals. If the baby is strong and over three months old, grated apple is also suitable: grate a quarter of a good apple on a glass or plastic grater and feed with a spoon. Then grate the next quarter, and so on. This can also be given for five meals for at least two days during which all other food, even rusks, is strictly omitted. After the second day just over 1 oz (30g) of the apple or carrot remedy is replaced by rice or oat gruel at each meal, after which there is a gradual transition back to normal food. At the earliest on the third day a dessertspoon of milk can be added to the meal. After this you may for some weeks have to resort to a pulverized baby food prescribed by the doctor.

Constipation

It was mentioned earlier that bottle-fed babies have firmer stools than breastfed children. Usually this is no cause for concern. Only if fewer than three stools are passed per week can one speak of constipation. In the case of bottle-fed babies a slight increase in fluid amounts is usually enough. If necessary one can also add small quantities of honey or lactose (1 level teaspoon spread over one day) to the feed. The breastfed baby will benefit from the mother drinking Weleda's Milk Forming Tea.

Until the whole digestion process has settled, one may need to help a bit with small enemas, using camomile tea at body temperature, but please consult a doctor for the best method of doing this. Laxatives not prescribed by a doctor should never be used!

In older children—especially girls—constipation is often a failure to empty the bowel regularly. This may be due to embarrassment or 'missing the moment'.

For chronic constipation there are additional dietary ways of stimulating natural elimination forces. Drinking a couple of mouthfuls of water in the morning on an empty stomach, or eating an apple, can help. In the evening, before going to sleep, a few dried prunes, softened in water, can be given. One can add wheatbran to breakfast or the evening meal, or drink herb tea sweetened with lactose. Linseed bread, honey cake and rye crackers are also helpful. If these natural means do not stimulate the bowel, a doctor should be consulted.

Vomiting

Vomiting is in itself not an illness but rather an often rather dramatic symptom of an incipient or acute disorder.

There are, however, forms of vomiting caused by the nervous system. This is sudden and violent and indicates brain disease. Usually, however, vomiting is simply a sign of an upset stomach as a result of wrong feeding. The doctor will need to know whether the baby's tongue is clean or coated and whether there is diarrhoea as well as vomiting.

With ketotic vomiting the baby's mouth smells faintly of apples or acetone. This is a form of vomiting that can easily recur and must be treated by the doctor. He will prescribe enemas of sugar water, and perhaps ipecacuanha which is given orally drop by drop. If the child is given anything to drink he will immediately vomit again.

Pyloric spasm is another form of vomiting that occurs in very young babies. It is a cramp of the muscle at the exit of the stomach which prevents the food from passing into the intestines, causing it instead to be violently vomited. Babies with this complaint are hard to feed. Best of all is the mother's milk given by teaspoon. There are also good natural remedies, but if nothing helps, the doctor may have to send the baby to hospital. It is often possible to recognize babies with a tendency to this problem soon after birth by the tense expression on their faces, their nerviness and deep horizontal frowns on the forehead. I have noticed that babies whose mothers had been unable to come to terms with their pregnancy or who had been suffering from depression at the onset of pregnancy tend towards this complaint.

There are also children who have a virtuoso skill in the art of vomiting and use this ability to tyrannize their anxious parents. Babies and children also vomit if forced to eat more than they need. Older children also vomit out of fear of exams or other events at school or at home. Unsuitable medicines, or actual poisons, also cause vomiting. And finally the nervous strain imposed by television watching has also now been recognized as a cause of vomiting.

Teething

Since the days of the ancient Greek physician Hippocrates there has been discussion of the symptoms of illness that occur in conjunction with the appearance of the first teeth. All mothers will have observed that before cutting a tooth the baby may refuse solid food, have diarrhoea, have a temperature of 101.3°F (38.5°C) or more, or show that their gums are tender by cramming their fists into their mouths, and of course crying. Some babies even start to cough, others suffer cramps, and when the eye-teeth come through they even sometimes contract conjunctivitis. The symptoms usually vanish as soon as the tooth is cut, and there is not a great deal that the doctor can do.

The cutting of the teeth, which are after all the hardest part of the whole organism, is a trial of strength for the whole human being. Vitamin B, especially B_6, can sometimes help to alleviate teething symptoms.

There is a wide variety of timing in teeth. In some families they come early, in others late. Rickets can cause exceptionally late teething, while some babies, for instance Napoleon, are born with teeth.

Usually children have four to six teeth by the beginning of their second year. As a rule of thumb we could say: In the sixth to ninth month the two middle lower incisors are cut; in the seventh to tenth month the four upper incisors; in the twelfth to fifteenth month the first upper molar on either side followed by the second pair of lower incisors, followed by the first lower molars; in the eighteenth to twenty-fourth month first the upper eye-teeth followed by the lower eye-teeth; in the thirtieth to thirty-sixth month finally the second pairs of molars appear, first the upper and then the lower.

Thus the milk teeth consist of eight incisors, eight molars and four eye-teeth, i.e. 20 teeth.

The second set of teeth, consisting usually of 32 teeth, starts to appear in the fifth or sixth year. It can be earlier or later but if it is much later the doctor should be consulted.

Usually a third pair of molars (top and bottom) appear. Then the milk teeth start to be pushed out, roughly in the order in which they came. Shortly before puberty the remaining canines appear, followed by the fourth pair of molars (upper and lower), and finally, sometimes many years later, the fifth pairs of molars (wisdom teeth).

The beginning of the change of teeth shows that the child has reached a certain degree of maturity, both physically and psychologically. Thus as a general rule a child whose milk teeth have not even started to wobble should if possible not be sent to school. Of course the falling out of rotten teeth cannot be regarded as a sign of maturity. Usually it is a sign of a faulty diet, though some children are simply afflicted with bad teeth.

Regular care of the teeth should start at 18 months. And even the milk teeth should be seen regularly by the dentist every six months.

Chills

Just as poison enters the organism via the mouth and stomach, so cold air can invade the organism through an exposed part of the skin, or through the mucous respiratory passages, the intestines, the bladder, the ears or eyes.

The result is a chill, which can afflict any part of the body, for instance as a cold in the nose, bronchitis, sinusitis, lumbago or flu. The ego is not working properly at the spot where the chill takes hold, and consequently disturbances arise in the organ which create favourable conditions for all sorts of agents that cause illness. These agents are thus not the primary cause but rather the consequence of the actual illness, but they bring about a worsening or spreading of the illness.

A useful remedy for a cold in the head region is a foot bath or even a full bath in which the heat of the water is gradually increased. (Footbaths with built in heater and thermostat are available on the market.) A sweat compress may also suffice (see page 187.)

A herbal tea is a good additional remedy, for instance a mixture of equal amounts of peppermint, fennel and camomile, or great mullein, coltsfoot, icelandic moss and camomile with a large teaspoon of honey. The latter must be added to the tea when it is ready to drink but not hotter than 104°F (40°C), as otherwise the life forces of the honey are destroyed. These teas are sipped by the patient. Sytra Tea (Weleda) is good for a cough.

Another useful traditional remedy: Boil two large onions in $\frac{3}{4}$ of a litre of water for one hour, sieve and add honey as above. Give the patient 1 to 2 dessertspoons every two hours.

For a more advanced cold or chill, a Schlenz Bath can be a great help (see pages 190–3). Thus a great deal can be done to relieve colds and chills.

Abdominal pain and gastro-intestinal complaints

Children suffer abdominal pains for a variety of reasons, most of which are harmless. Some, however, must be taken seriously, so the doctor should be consulted if the pain lasts for more than an hour, especially if the child feels sick or actually does vomit. Take the child's temperature under the arm and in the rectum (each five minutes) and inform the doctor of both readings over the phone (see page 180).

Sometimes the pains are caused by the food the child eats,

either because he has eaten too much or because the food is of poor quality or made unpalatable by chemical additives.

However, the possibility of appendicitis or something similar must always be borne in mind, since even small babies can have appendicitis, though this is more likely with babies fed on commercial baby foods. Children can also contract stomach ulcers, a consequence of the so-called 'civilized' foods of today with their predominance of sugar and white flour. Inflammation of the gall bladder and also jaundice are no longer rare, whereas 40 years ago it was most unusual for a child to suffer from a liver or gall bladder complaint.

Usually abdominal pain, vomiting and diarrhoea are indications of poisoning or an intestinal problem, especially if the child has shivering fits, a headache and a dry or coated tongue.

With food poisoning usually all those who have eaten the contaminated dish are affected. But with gastroenteritis members of a family usually take it in turns to succumb. There is always a possibility of typhoid, especially in hot weather.

Small children usually complain of abdominal pain when they have a sore throat, especially in the early stages of the attack.

Newborn and small infants often suffer from wind and abdominal pain when breastfed if the mother is too restless, anxious or agitated, or if she eats too much raw fruit, or drinks coffee or strong tea.

Abdominal cramps (colic) every few minutes interspersed with pain-free intervals followed by constipation and vomiting point to the possibility of a twisting of the intestines. This can occur in children as young as four months.

Either the intestine is blocked by twisting into a loop, or the upper end of the intestines pushes itself into the lower part. (I have seen a case where the small intestine had passed right through the large intestine and protruded for about 10 centimetres from the rectum.) If such possibilities are borne in mind, preventive measures can be taken before it is too late, so consult the doctor in good time!

Children with poor appetites often have 'tummy ache' before or during every meal from dread of the daily torture of being forced to eat. It is quite wrong to force unwilling children to eat, since this causes cramps in stomach or intestines which make the digestive glands cease the secretion of digestive juices, resulting in actual inability to digest the unwelcome food.

Other children get tummy ache if they dread going to school or are afflicted with other anxieties. Happy excitement, for instance looking forward to a journey, can also cause painful cramps in the digestive organs. In fact excitement of all kinds can cause 'stomach cramps', diarrhoea or vomiting.

Chemical medicaments, worm cures or laxatives can cause intestinal allergies leading to painful irritation of the intestinal mucous membranes. Fresh bread and also vegetables, especially spinach, grown with artificial fertilizer can all cause painful intestinal conditions. Intestinal tuberculosis, which is very rare nowadays, causes similar symptoms. Even grapes not properly washed (first briefly in hot and then in cold water) and other sprayed fruit eaten with its skin can cause serious symptoms.

The doctor should always be consulted, especially if the symptoms keep recurring, and if the mother knows the various possibilities she will be able to make valuable observations that can help the doctor in his diagnosis.

In obvious cases of cramp or colic, when there is no likelihood of appendicitis, relief can be obtained by applying a warmed bag of camomile flowers or hayflowers (flores graminis) to the abdomen (see page 189).

Appendicitis

The danger with an inflammation of the appendix and the neighbouring intestine is that it might become perforated, allowing the contents of the intestine to spill into the abdominal cavity, causing peritonitis. Perforation can occur quite quickly, only a few hours after the onset of the abdominal pains, or it does not occur at all, which is usually the case.

Until quite recently every inflamed appendix was immediately removed, although in about 80 per cent of the cases the appendix itself was found to be not at all or only slightly inflamed. It was considered to be a superfluous organ that might have had some function during earlier phases of human evolution. Nowadays it has become apparent that it may not be as unimportant as had been thought but may have to do with the secretion of lymph active in increasing resistance to infections. I have rarely found it necessary to have an appendix operated. But diagnosis is very difficult as the symptoms are so varied. There may be virtually no pain, or no temperature. And when there is doubt, the patient should have the operation without delay. Even tiny babies can have acute inflammation of the appendix.

If a child suddenly stops playing and complains of tummy

ache and feeling sick, he should be put to bed immediately. All inflammation needs peace and quiet and the child should be persuaded to lie as still as possible. If necessary his legs can be tied together with a scarf or nappy. After 20 minutes lying quietly the temperature can be taken (see *Taking the temperature*, pages 180–1). Give absolutely *nothing* to eat or drink.

If the discomfort continues (sharp pains on the right side of the abdomen, first higher up and later lower down, feeling sick or vomiting, rapid pulse, an ailing demeanour and tense facial expression) the doctor should be called immediately, even in the middle of the night. Tell him the two temperature measurements (see page 181).

If the intestine is empty as a result of the child being given no food or drink, there is far less likelihood of perforation of the appendix. A small, gentle (balloon) enema can be given to clear the intestine, but on no account any laxative or laxative tea. The enema consists of no more than a little cool water. On no account should warm compresses be applied to the abdomen. The doctor will decide whether cold or other compresses should be applied.

If there is no need for an operation, which is usually the case, medicinal treatment can be allowed to come into its own. There are anthroposophical and similar medicines and methods which can combat even acute appendicitis, and it is a serious mistake to believe that only antibiotics are suitable.

Pneumonia

A heavy cold, especially if it results from an attack of flu, can easily turn into pneumonia, particularly if a medicine has been given to suppress rather than loosen the cough. For

instance with measles there is hardly likely to be a complication of pneumonia if the cough has not been suppressed
with medicines containing codeine.

Pneumonia may be recognized by the high temperature,
the agitation of the child, the shallow breathing often
accompanied by moaning, and the way the nostrils dilate
every time a breath is exhaled. The child also has a very red
face and often feels sharp pains in the chest. If the inflammation is just beginning, all these symptoms will be slight.
The pain is not in the lungs but in the pleura or bronchial
tubes.

In my experience, treatment with antibiotics is not
necessary. I have always achieved perfect recovery without
them. My aim is not to suppress the course of the illness but
to help the patient while it runs its course. Without a doubt
children who are helped through the illness in this way gain
new and valuable capacities that help them to master life. If
pneumonia is suspected, the doctor must be called immediately. He may prescribe compresses (see pages 187–8).

Croup and diphtheria

Croup arises when there is a sudden swelling of the mucous
membranes deep down in the throat and in the larynx, which
can lead to a narrowing of the windpipe almost causing
suffocation. The cough is dry and barking. The condition
looks more alarming than it is, and if the mother keeps calm
and does not excite the child, causing him to breathe ir-
regularly, he will be able to get enough breath. So even if the
first attack comes in the middle of the night and looks very
alarming, keep calm! Try immediately to make the air in the

bedroom as damp as possible, for instance by boiling an electric kettle. Or take the child into the bathroom and let hot water run into the bath, so that the child can breathe in the steam. Then put the child back to bed with the upper part of his body raised to ease his breathing.

Attacks of this kind usually occur at the beginning of winter or in February or March. They are without fever unless they are complicated by bronchitis or something similar. Usually the child will have been perfectly healthy during the day and then suddenly at about nine o'clock at night will be woken by the loud barking cough. The pattern will be repeated during the following evenings if the doctor has not succeeded in taking suitable measures. There are natural remedies which are very effective, and the doctor may also recommend hot compresses (see pages 187–9). Children who have been overfed with milk or other foods are prone to these attacks of croup.

In contrast, diphtheria is dangerous, because the windpipe is coated with mucous. It is now very rare. The cough is a dry barking cough arising in the region of the larynx. It must not be confused with croup. Diphtheria is accompanied by a temperature, and a bad smell from the mouth. The doctor must verify the condition by an examination of the throat. The temperature with diphtheria is usually not more than 102.2°C (39°C), that is less than with flu or tonsillitis. The saliva and mucous expelled by the coughing are of course very infectious.

Inflammation of the middle ear

Inflammation of the middle ear can arise fairly easily as a complication of a bad cold or in particular of tonsillitis which has not been properly cured. With infants as well as older children it usually starts first at night with isolated sharp pain in the ear. The child wakes and cries. The following night the attacks are more frequent and the pain worse. Babies throw their head to and fro and rub the painful ear with their hand. There is also an acute form of the illness which sets in immediately with very bad pain.

The pain can often be soothed by pouring a few drops of warm milk or oil into the ear while pulling gently at the outer ear to help the liquid seep down to the ear drum while letting the air in the passage escape. (Method: Boil water and dip the bowl of a spoon into this to absorb the heat. Pour a few drops of sunflower, olive or Weleda silica oil into the spoon and wait for half a minute. The oil will then have the correct temperature for pouring into the ear.)

An onion poultice can help if the pain if very bad, as the onion draws the inflammation towards the outside (see page 194). But the doctor must be consulted.

Every domestic medicine chest should contain a paediatric analgesic for the relief of very bad pain.

If the child has a temperature, cold compresses on the calves can be applied to relieve the pressure of blood in the head, though not to completely dampen down the temperature. A sweat compress or Schlenz Bath is very important on the morning after a night of earache. In addition the doctor will prescribe one of the natural remedies that has proved successful for ear inflammation.

Lancing of the ear drum is only necessary in rare cases. If the ear drum bursts of its own accord, careful rinsing with camomile will assist the discharge of pus. See that the child lies on the sick ear to allow the rinse to drain away. The child will have to remain under the care of the doctor to ensure that the condition does not become chronic. If the condition worsens and develops into mastoid infection, even this can be cured in most cases by medical treatment. If this fails, there will have to be an operation to prevent the pus from making its way into the blood vessels of the brain.

Acute tonsillitis

The doctor must always be consulted when the tonsils are inflamed, since there are many forms of tonsillitis. The mother, for instance cannot distinguish between tonsillitis and diphtheria, and though the latter is a disease 'of the past' its pattern of recurrence is not known and one cannot be too careful. There are also other malignant forms of tonsillitis which may at first appear quite harmless.

The mother can support the work of the doctor by giving the child as little protein as possible, i.e. no meat or eggs, while giving instead fresh lemon, orange and raw vegetable juices. The digestion may need to be supported with a milk laxative or a laxative tea. Very small children can be given an enema.

Serious illness can often be averted by giving the child as soon as possible an intensive footbath (Schlenz Footbath, see page 192). For a throat compress, lemon is suitable. Make incisions all round half an unsprayed lemon under water in a bowl, then press the lemon against the bottom of the bowl, thus squeezing out the juice. (Half a lemon is sufficient for one compress.) If the lemon is sprayed, just squeeze the juice into the water without immersing the skin. If the nose is blocked, let the child inhale the steam from camomile tea.

An effective preventive measure: for about six weeks during the autumn wash the child's neck and upper trunk with sea-salt water daily.

Vaccination—Fundamental considerations

What is vaccination? In general, vaccination is carried out as a protection against certain infectious diseases. Infection is caused by the invasion of the organism by bacteria or viruses (or innumerable other agents or toxic substances) leading to the typical symptoms of the illness in question. Some examples are: pneumonia, pyelonephritis, typhoid fever, dysentery, lung tuberculosis, polio, venereal diseases, and also the childhood diseases discussed in this book.

A number of these illnesses, e.g. the childhood diseases, polio, tuberculosis, and (if the patient survives) smallpox and tetanus only attack an individual once. After the attack he is immune.

The explanation for this is that during an illness of this kind certain antibodies form in the blood of the afflicted person and annihilate the cause of the illness. These antibodies remain in the blood throughout life, preventing a new infection with the illness even if the person is in contact with others who are infected. The time it takes for the antibodies to form is called the immunization phase.

Other infectious illnesses such as pneumonia or flu do not result in permanent immunity. The antibodies disappear again after a while and the person can be infected anew.

A new step was taken when medical science learnt how to bring about immunization artificially. Jenner and Koch were pioneers in this. A weakened form of the cause of the disease was inoculated under the skin, thus causing a controlled infection.

Unfortunately the hopes raised by this new method have not been entirely fulfilled. This will be discussed in more detail.

First, however, let us briefly mention so-called passive vaccination. In this case, serum from the blood of animals containing the immunization substance is injected. This method is usually used where rapid protection is required. The best known of these is the anti-tetanus serum for injuries. In a similar way, though completely naturally, breastfed babies are protected during their early months because they imbibe antibodies with their mother's milk.

When a baby is subjected to active immunization, a powerful biological revolution takes place from which he takes a long time to recover. All the greater is the strain resulting from multiple vaccination. Threefold, fourfold and even fivefold vaccinations force me to conclude that the infant organism is regarded as an automaton into which any number of antigens can be introduced which then lead to the same number of immunities. This is an invasion of medicine by computer mentality.

It is high time to oppose this dangerous enthusiasm for vaccination, especially with vaccines (such as the fivefold vaccine) which have been insufficiently tested. Recently a child died two days after being treated with the fivefold vaccine. Also the assertion* that the first vaccination against smallpox should take place during the early months of life

---

* In a number of countries, including Britain, routine vaccination of small children against smallpox is no longer undertaken.

strikes me as being highly doubtful, especially as a considerable amount has been published asserting that this method is of little value. In recent years, more people have died in England from smallpox vaccination than from smallpox. For smallpox vaccination I strongly advise the new dry vaccine.

Over the years it has become evident that the attitude to vaccination in this book coincides with that of many specialists in the field. Professor Stickel, Director of the Munich Institute for Vaccination, for instance, warns against misuse and excessive use of vaccination. He suggests that smallpox vaccination, obviously only given to healthy children, should not be administered before the second year. 'Problem children', that is any child whose physical or psychological development is not normal, must not be vaccinated. No vaccination for measles. No multiple vaccinations. Tetanus vaccination not until the second or third year. And in general, vaccination should only be undertaken if it is really necessary.

Gynaecologists, furthermore, state that smallpox vaccination should be avoided throughout pregnancy, because of the danger to the child. Small children should also not be vaccinated if their mother is pregnant again.

The fact that, despite all this, the vaccination of babies and infants persists, comes about because they show very little reaction, whereas older children can react with cramps, fever, vomiting and confusion. It is now known that small children react so mildly because they do not yet possess sufficient strength with which to counteract the vaccination. Thus the danger is all the greater that the vaccine will affect the brain. In the embryo, the skin and the membranes of the brain develop from the same germ cell. Thus all vaccinations applied in or under the skin (smallpox, tuberculosis, whooping cough, measles, etc.) can easily affect the brain.

A further risk is presented by multiple vaccinations or by single vaccinations administered at short intervals. After a vaccination, during the immunization phase (see above), the patient is busy reacting to one particular vaccination and is therefore not able to react to others (see below).

It is essential to realize, furthermore, that immunity does not last a lifetime, whereas an attack of a childhood disease in the natural way does lead to lifelong immunity. In most cases protection through vaccination lasts only for a few years. Hence the many repeat vaccinations that are necessary, for instance for smallpox, measles, polio etc. And hence also the danger of the child contracting the disease despite the vaccination. When this happens the illness is usually particularly serious and dangerous. These children obviously have little capacity to react out of themselves.

It is obvious that the vaccination question requires a great deal of responsible consideration. Every case is different and must be considered individually. All fanatical advertising in favour of vaccination should be condemned, especially as it usually engenders excessive fear.

In the United States, where there has for years been no case of smallpox but where there have been numerous cases of damage from vaccination, the abolition of smallpox vaccination is being considered. Similarly in Japan. In Germany, smallpox vaccination is no longer compulsory (since 1976), except in certain cases: re-vaccination of twelve-year-olds who were vaccinated as small children, for certain professions, and if there is a danger of infection. It is felt by the authorities that the abolition of compulsion is justified on the ground of the success of the World Health Organization's programme to eradicate the disease. This sensible decision has, furthermore, surely come about from the realization that the advantages have been exaggerated in relation to the tragic damage (and the resulting costs) that can ensue.

Epidemics are as unpredictable as the weather; our knowledge of their laws is full of gaps. It seems to me that we should not rely too much on statistics nor place too much confidence in vaccination alone.

Since the introduction of oral vaccination the incidence of polio has dwindled to a few isolated cases; certainly cases of paralysis and death hardly occur any more. However, I doubt whether the prevention of paralysis really means that the polio problem can be regarded as overcome. Diphtheria is an equally dangerous illness which has at present become rare. Yet nobody can seriously maintain that the relatively small proportion of diphtheria vaccinations is the cause of this reduction; in fact the disease began to dwindle before the diphtheria serum was even invented. Epidemics of plague, cholera, typhus and spotted fever have 'disappeared' from the civilized world without any vaccination, perhaps because of improved hygienic conditions. But is this the only explanation? In my opinion there are other aspects to consider in relation to illness and epidemics in addition to the fact that they are caused by bacteria or viruses.

The four parts of the human being—physical body, life forces, soul forces and spiritual forces—have been mentioned a number of times in this book. I would like to maintain that when these four members are in harmony, infections are warded off or overcome. Only when they are in disharmony can infections take hold. This applies even more to the virus infections which threaten us today than to the bacterial epidemics of the past. It must be admitted that the pressures of life today lead to considerable disturbances of the interplay between man's four members and from this point of view it would seem that there is no lack of opportunity for virus infections to take hold.

Vaccination, however, is not the only protection. Professor Pette, a well-known vaccination expert and neurologist, wrote a few years ago: 'Every vaccination is a serious interference with the human organism.' This throws light on the fact that the general standard of health in countries which undertake a great deal of vaccination is considerably lower than in countries which have approached vaccination with more hesitation. Of course there are also other causes for this phenomenon, but it nevertheless gives cause for concern.

Even if it turns out in the end that vaccination does give proper protection to the individual, there are a number of grave objections to its use. In some countries infants receive as many as 14 injections in the first three months of life and the number is likely to increase as new vaccines are discovered. Doctors who include all four aspects of the human being in their considerations cannot but be exceedingly worried by this prospect. It seems extremely likely that the general resistance to illness of those vaccinated will decrease progressively, that their ability to stand up to stress will decrease, and that sterility, allergies and above all liver damage will result from increased vaccination. This is already becoming apparent in the poor health standards of those countries with the most comprehensive vaccination programmes.

Another serious objection to vaccination is that it obscures the real reasons for the increasing incidence of new virus infections. Since reforms are always unpopular, we shall no doubt continue to live unhealthy lives, making light of malnutrition arising from poor food quality, persisting in overstimulating our nervous systems, and turning to the panacea of the latest vaccine whenever we need it.

The illusion that we can drag from the earth unlimited supplies of food if only we put back enough mineral fertilizers and kill enough pests with chemical sprays seems to me similar to the illusion that we can continue indefinitely to combat illness with vaccination.

However, I must stress that I do not want to prevent anyone from having himself or his children vaccinated. Particularly with polio it has been shown that fear increases the chances of contracting the disease. It cannot be my business to prevent anyone from accepting vaccination. So far, for instance, oral vaccination against polio seems to be a complete success. Nevertheless, this was also thought to be the case with smallpox vaccination until experience gave rise to doubts. So let us not rely too heavily on vaccination, which may turn out to be an illusion based on wishful thinking. Instead let us do all we can to increase the body's natural resistance to epidemics. There are plenty of suggestions in this book of ways to do this.

Frequent questions about vaccination

- *In the case of oral vaccination against polio is there any danger of the virus being transferred to unvaccinated persons?*
  Experience has shown that the amount of virus which may

pass from treated to untreated persons is not enough to cause an infection. It is conceivable that in the case of a small child receiving this vaccination, others in the same household might be infected but so far this has not been known to happen. Of course extra cleanliness must be observed, especially in dealing with the nappy or potty of the child.

- *Who should definitely not be vaccinated?*
Anyone suffering from an acute illness with or without fever; anyone with a stomach or intestinal complaint (diarrhoea, gastritis, enteritis, etc.); anyone undergoing a course of treatment with cortisone; anyone with one of the infectious children's diseases. For smallpox vaccination the patient's skin must in addition be absolutely healthy. For vaccination in pregnancy see below.

- *How much time must elapse between vaccinations?*
After a first vaccination against smallpox, and after subsequent vaccinations if pustules have appeared, at least six weeks must elapse before other vaccinations are undertaken. If in the case of second or subsequent vaccinations only a small lump appears, other vaccinations can be undertaken after a week.

After BCG vaccination against tuberculosis at least three months must elapse before a first smallpox vaccination is undertaken. After oral vaccination against polio and after yellow fever vaccination four weeks must elapse before a smallpox vaccination is undertaken. A three-week gap is sufficient after other vaccinations.

If tetanus serum or other animal serum (horse, cow or sheep) has been injected, three weeks must elapse before smallpox vaccination is undertaken.

Vaccination during pregnancy

In the first three months all vaccination must be avoided, especially polio and smallpox. If at all possible it should be avoided during the whole of pregnancy, even if needed for foreign travel.

The virus in smallpox vaccination can pass from the blood of the expectant mother to that of the baby. This is all the more reason to avoid it during pregnancy, especially in the first three and in the final months. For the same reason oral vaccination with live virus against polio should be avoided, especially during the early months. Treatment with BCG vaccine against tuberculosis is only recommended if the expectant mother has unavoidable, close contact with a patient suffering from open tuberculosis where isolation is impossible.

Important note on vaccination

For every vaccination give the person Weleda Thuja 30x drops starting on the day of the vaccination (3–5 drops morning and evening on an empty stomach). For smallpox vaccination continue till the pustules have disappeared.

Fever resulting from vaccination can lead to brain damage and the use of Thuja 30x with every vaccination helps protect the brain.

3. CHILDHOOD ILLNESSES

Many of the so-called childhood illnesses, many of which have grown rarer due to vaccination, have often been observed to enhance a child's development. Following such an illness the child will frequently seem more present and dexterous in his body, and more alert in soul. The accompanying fever helps the ego incarnate more fully, and at the same time the natural occurrence of these illnesses, unlike vaccination, gives lifelong immunity against their recurrence. The childhood illnesses are almost invariably far more serious, and even dangerous, when they occur in adolescence and adulthood.

Incubation periods and duration of infectiousness

	Incubation period	Duration of infectiousness
Diphtheria	2–7 days	Patient is no longer infectious after the third negative throat and nose swab
Whooping cough	8–21 days	When the whooping stops
Measles	9–11 days	After three weeks
Polio★	8–14 days	Isolation usually 6 weeks
Mumps	16–22 days	Patient is no longer infectious when all symptoms have disappeared
Scarlet fever	1–7 days	Isolation usually 6 weeks
Chickenpox	2–3 weeks	Patient no longer infectious after 3 weeks
German measles	2–3 weeks	Patient no longer infectious after 10 days

★ Polio and some virus diseases are only infectious in exceptional circumstances.

Measles

With the childhood illnesses which share the symptom of a red rash (measles, scarlet fever, German measles) the purpose of the illness is particularly clear. Most children need measles for their healthy development and are thus 'inwardly prepared' for the illness. This is why they nearly always catch the disease if they contact infection. Before vaccination against it became common, it used to be quite an exception not to have gone through measles. Even brief contact with a patient in the infectious stage, especially in the days before the rash appears, will lead in ten or eleven days to the onset of the initial catarrh, followed in three or four days by the outbreak of the rash. The picture painted by the rash on the child's skin reveals the nature of this illness. As the temperature rises, the facial skin swells, making the features indistinct. The mucous membranes of the eyes, nose, throat, larynx and windpipe are also swollen and inflamed and show a liquid discharge. Starting behind the ears a patchy red rash spreads over the head and then over the whole body as well as the internal mucous membranes. The child develops conjunctivitis, avoids the light, and has a cold in the nose and catarrh in the respiratory passages. Not infrequently the pressure on the brain increases, with consequent cramps or disturbances of consciousness. The white spots which appear inside the cheeks identify measles finally, since it is not often easy to distinguish the rash from that of German measles.

After three or four days the rash fades, the facial swelling recedes, the inflammation of the mucous membranes diminishes, the cough and cold cease, and the child recovers rapidly. There are, however, cases in which the cough is very bad and persistent and the child feels very ill for quite some time.

The following remarks may help in the treatment and nursing of measles: All unnecessary treatment should be avoided. In particular the temperature should not be suppressed, even if it exceeds 104°F (40°C). Similarly the cough must not be suppressed. Such measures can lead to justifiably dreaded pneumonia arising as a complication of measles. The inflamed state of the mucous membranes leads unavoidably to considerable coughing. Weleda Cough Elixir is a good loosener and brings relief. Nothing much more need be done, as the cough will diminish after two or three days anyway. No chest compresses should be applied while the rash is visible. If the child is very restless he can be given a quick wipe with vinegar water. To avoid cooling off, work quickly and rub energetically all over the trunk and legs with a mixture of two thirds lukewarm water and one third wine or cider vinegar. Do not dry. If the child avoids light the room should be darkened. The bowel must be moved daily, if necessary with the help of an enema. The diet should consist above all of fruit juice and fresh fruit, or with small children hot milk diluted half and half with mineral water. No protein-rich, so-called 'nourishing' food should be given and the return to a normal diet should not start till the child demands it. The child must stay in bed for ten days and have a further ten to 14 days quiet at home. When the fever has abated, Weleda Waldon II is a good tonic, but so are a number of natural calcium preparations with additional iron.

Scarlet fever

Scarlet fever is much more uncommon than measles, and serious cases are now rare. In contrast to measles, though, even light cases of scarlet fever must be taken seriously, especially the 'second phase' of the illness, which usually starts during the third week, since there is a danger of complications involving the kidneys or ears. Scarlet fever is far less infectious than measles, but the contagion is erratic, so strict isolation is necessary for six weeks.

The illness usually starts suddenly without much preliminary discomfort. The initial symptoms are high temperature, vomiting, headache, and in small children sometimes convulsions. Soon the tonsils become inflamed and the soft palate turns a flaming red. The itchy rash appears on the very first day, on the neck and then spreading over the whole torso. The thickly clustered minute red spots gradually merge to make a uniform redness of the skin. Quite often, however, the rash hardly develops and can only be detected by careful scrutiny of the groin and the inside of the thighs. Thus it is frequently overlooked. Diagnosis is helped by the strawberry tongue which appears after three or four days. After about five days, the skin redness gradually fades. In the second or third week the outer skin begins to peel, first in small flakes but later often in large shreds. There are a number of feverish illnesses accompanied by rashes that resemble that of scarlet fever. In some cases final diagnosis is only possible when the skin starts to peel.

The doctor must definitely be consulted when the child has scarlet fever, but the modern rapid cure with antibiotics should be avoided if at all possible.

During the first five or six days the child is given only fruit juice or raw fruit, until the tongue is clean again. Daily bowel movement is assured with the help of Weleda Clairo Tea or if necessary with an enema. If the constipation is very solid, a camomile enema can be given. The child must be kept strictly in bed even in the third week, since this is the point when the ears or kidneys can become affected.

Chickenpox

Chickenpox is extremely infectious. The child does not have a very high temperature. The rash consists of tiny watery blisters covering the whole body, including the scalp, the inside of the mouth and the mucous membranes of eyes, ears and genitals. They last for about five days, during which some heal while new ones continue to appear. Sometimes the patient has only a few of these blisters, while in other epidemics the body is covered with hundreds of them. The rash is extremely irritating, and if it is extensive the child must be kept in bed for a few days. If scratched, the blisters will leave small scars. To relieve the itching, dab the places with vinegar water ($\frac{2}{3}$ water, $\frac{1}{3}$ vinegar) and afterwards sprinkle with powder.

German measles

This is such a mild illness that it hardly needs any treatment, except perhaps the many lymph gland swellings, particularly on the back of the neck. Strict isolation is unnecessary, and the child can return to school after ten days. Lifelong immunity is assured. The rash sometimes resembles a light attack of measles, at others it is more like that of scarlet fever. (Regarding German measles in pregnancy, see pages 13–14.)

Mumps

Mumps is a virus infection. Infection usually takes place from person to person, more rarely via healthy carriers, and most rarely via infected objects. It is a very infectious disease, except that small babies do not so easily catch it. It is rare for a person to have the illness more than once. In recent years it has become more serious than it used to be.

The temperature is usually high for a short time. The parotid salivary gland in the neck swells, often on one side at a time, and is painful when pressed. Chewing is painful, and the ear can hurt. Sometimes the submandibular salivary gland is also affected. Complications can be inflammation of the scrotum and also meningitis, but this is unusual before puberty.

Treatment should not be taken lightly. If the child has a temperature he should be kept in bed, preferably for too long rather than too short a time. Let him rinse his mouth and gargle with sage tea or Weleda Mouth Wash and make sure his bowel movements are adequate. The swollen glands may be covered with cotton wool soaked in hot oil or with an ointment prescribed by the doctor. The diet should be vegetarian with plenty of fruit and as little protein as possible.

Whooping cough

Many doctors still regard this illness as a threat to the life of babies and small children. Certainly in the past thousands of children did die of it every year and deaths do still occur occasionally.

More than with any other illness it is now possible to prove the superior efficacy of natural remedies and methods. Treated in this way, no otherwise healthy child, or even small baby, dies of whooping cough today. The complications of this illness, which usually involve the brain, are also avoided with these methods.

The main innovation is that the whooping attacks are not suppressed but rather helped to take place, while the cramp is loosened to the extent of no longer being dangerous.

Preventive vaccination should be avoided, for whooping cough is most certainly a 'healthy disease'.

Of course this is not to say that the mother will not have a good many disturbed nights. But the attacks look worse than they are, which becomes obvious when you see the child resume playing happily as soon as the attack is over. Sensible parents will come to terms with even the heavy attacks, which occur for a duration of eight to ten days, when they understand that this is a crisis which will have a favourable outcome. (Lighter attacks may go on for much longer.) If the parents overcome their worries, the atmosphere in the house will be free from anxiety. When the child has an attack, encourage him not to worry and let him spit out the catarrh or even vomit his recent meal. After the attack, first give the child his medicine and then a small snack. Thus food is not taken at the normal mealtimes but little by little after each attack. It should be light, in small portions and without crumbs which might unnecessarily stimulate a new attack of coughing. Children who do not eat much usually pass through the coughing phase particularly rapidly. Some loss of weight is of no account, since the child's subsequent excellent appetite will soon put this right.

The medicine that has achieved the success described above is Pertudoron I and II (Weleda). The doctor will advise about the dosage, but do not give it too frequently.

The course of the illness can be complicated by bronchitis or some other acute attacks.

Apart from a light and sparse diet, the mother can also help the child considerably by remaining absolutely calm. The room may be aired after each attack. While the attacks are at their most violent, there is no point in taking the child out into the open air. Rapid movements bring on attacks. Cold wind, especially east wind, is particularly unsuitable. Relief can also be given with hot chest poultices or compresses with warm beeswax for ten minutes (see pages 193–4). It is superfluous to travel with the child for the sake of a change of air. It unnecessarily spreads the infection to other children and a change of air can sometimes make the attacks worse. In some cases a flight lasting an hour during which an altitude of 3000 metres is maintained for at least 20 minutes can help to alleviate attacks. But this can frighten the child, which is of course counterproductive.

Parents and especially grandparents can catch whooping cough from the children. Adults will suffer from a persistent, violent cough, especially in the morning. Pertudoron is of great help to adults too, and they should start to take it at the first sign, though not more frequently than at two-hour intervals, taking the drops alternately. The number of drops varies according to the age of the patient.

Polio

As a result of the widespread use of oral vaccination against
polio, this disease is at the moment on the wane. But to assist
an early diagnosis, should it occur, the following description
is included.

The illness usually starts with a feverish attack of one kind
or another (a cold, flu, bronchitis, acute diarrhoea, middle ear
infection, tonsillitis, etc.). Then the temperature goes down
for one or several days, after which it rises again. This is
accompanied by bad headaches and pain in the spine, particularly in the loins, spreading into the abdomen and thighs.
Nearly always there is also pain and stiffness in the neck. The
doctor must be consulted immediately.

In all feverish illnesses, including polio, children should be
kept very quiet in bed for several days after the first onset of
fever. If polio is suspected it is essential to keep the patient
very still in bed. In the USA it is recommended that children
be left at home in less severe cases. If the child has to go to
hospital he should be carried to the ambulance rather than
walking. In severe cases and in all cases involving breathing
disturbances, the child must be admitted to hospital. Severe
paralysis can often improve in a few days through the medical
treatment described below.

Before admission to hospital an injection of Skorodit
(arsenic-iron compound) should be given by the doctor,
which usually halts the spread of paralysis to other groups of
muscles.

Fever-inhibiting and all other synthetic medicines must
be avoided at all costs. The fever is necessary for healing,
and as long as the fever persists, the chances of a cure are

good. If there is severe pain an analgesic will be unavoid-able.

As soon as polio is suspected, but also where paralysis has already manifested, soda compresses are very helpful: place a folded cloth in two pints (1 litre) of very hot water and add a heaped teaspoon of ordinary soda. Wring out this cloth in a dry towel and place it steaming under the patient's painful spine, without making him sit up. Renew the compress once it starts to cool. Alternatively, place the child in a soda bath, supporting his head well so that he doesn't have to actively keep it upright. A heaped dessertspoon (30g) of soda is added to the bathwater. The water should be body temperature to begin with, then pour in hot water after ten minutes until it reaches 39 degrees Celsius. One bath is given per day, lasting ten to 20 minutes, using the fever thermometer, as bath thermometers are not precise enough. However these soda baths should not be given if there is any sign at all of breathing difficulties. The compresses can be given two to three times a day.

I can only speak in general here about medical treatment, which is an area for the doctor. Since polio is a complex illness, therapy involves several mutually enhancing medi-cines.

An important task for the mother or nurse is to carry out the essential placing of the paralysed limbs as prescribed by the doctor. This applies particularly to the careful positioning of the upper arms and the feet, which must be placed against a solid board to avoid a pointed foot position.

One only starts with massage once the pain in muscles and nerves has abated. The patient can gradually and carefully attempt movement once the spread of pain has stopped.

Later, active, ongoing exercises are of the greatest importance, including perhaps physiotherapy.

One preventive measure against polio is to ensure a
wholesome diet. It has been found that polio often occurs in
people with insufficient bacterial flora in the intestines.
Refined carbohydrates and sugars should therefore be
avoided. Apart from fresh fruit, vegetables and live yoghurt,
garlic and oats are particularly beneficial.

In the case of a suspected infection, ensure regular bowel
movements, where necessary with a laxative tea (Weleda
Clairo Tea or similar). Also ensure absolute cleanliness. The
toilet and all enema equipment should be regularly disin-
fected with soda. Do not use any chemical disinfectants!
Avoid all physical exertion, especially in hot weather, and
direct sunlight.

Operations and vaccinations should also be avoided.

4. CHRONIC ILLNESSES

Hearing defects

If a child shows no reactions to noise in his second year, or if
he has shown no signs of starting to speak by the time he is 18
months old, hearing problems must be suspected.

During the past 20 years the number of children with
hearing problems seems to have increased. This may be
connected with the increase of loud noise in our environment. Deafness can also follow from chickenpox.

However, much progress has also been made in the
treatment of even severe deafness in children. The earlier the
problem is discovered the better. Hearing aids can now

utilize even the smallest remnants of hearing ability, thus making it possible for severely deaf children to learn to speak. Children with deafness in the family should be examined as early as possible, certainly long before they go to school.

Sight defects

Normally the proper functioning of the eyes is not achieved till the fourth or fifth year. The child only learns gradually to understand the sight impressions he receives daily from the moment of birth. Thus it is quite normal for a one-year old to look at a picture book upside down, to miss an object he is reaching for, or to try to touch the moon. On the other hand there is a great danger that sight disturbances (for instance short or long sight, colour blindness, or even congenital blindness) are overlooked or discovered too late. In families who suffer from these problems they are more likely to be noticed.

Anything unusual should be reported to the doctor, for instance lack of expression, either of joy or sorrow, in the eyes, or lack of reaction in the pupils. These decrease in bright light or on looking into the distance and increase in poor light or when the eyes are closed; other stimuli, such as pain or noise, cause the pupils to change as well. Large pupils can be a sign of short-sightedness and small pupils of long-sightedness. There may also be unusual movements of the eyeballs, such as trembling or twitching.

Congenital squinting is more common. It can be caused by disturbances in the balance of the eye muscles or by paralysis of some of those muscles. Medical treatment is necessary.

Since the child grasps his surroundings in the first place

through his eyes, it is most important to make sure that he is seeing a clear and not a clouded picture (long or short sight), and a single rather than a double image (squinting). It is obvious that someone seeing a distorted world will be a prey to psychological disturbances and be unable to think clearly.

There are many ways in which the doctor can help in these problems, starting with spectacles, which need not be a cause for distress.

Speech disorders

Children speak in an immediate flow that one should not interrupt unnecessarily with corrections, since they may then lose their immediacy of expression, and speech disorders could possibly ensue.

All children make 'mistakes' in their speech, stumbling over words or speaking words wrongly. Mostly these are related to their temperament and vanish naturally in the course of time. It is therefore not a good idea to draw children's attention to such errors by continually correcting them. The best remedy is for parents and teachers to speak clearly themselves, and to exclude unnecessary excitement such as TV. Television has actually been shown to delay speech development in children.

This is also the best approach in the case of lisping, stammering or stuttering etc. It is wrong to believe that one can remedy such disorders at a young age with intensive speech exercises. Rather, good speech develops on the basis of good physical movement. Children with a speech disorder should therefore play and move as much as possible, do eurythmy therapy, sing, and speak poems.

If speech disorders continue beyond the ninth year, speech therapy may be called for.

Lack of appetite

Children with chronically poor appetite are usually pale, anaemic, thin and tire easily. Their muscles are slack, their digestion disturbed, their body size is larger than normal but their weight is less than it should be. Such children are restless, fidgety and complain of sudden stomach pains. Often their mood fluctuates a good deal, their soul forces are directed too much on the external world whereas they should really be still active in the body's synthesizing organs.

The cure must depend on interesting these children's soul forces in the synthesizing metabolism once more.

This can occur, for instance, by administering the bitter substances of the gentian root. It is remarkable how willingly these children take medicines such as Weleda's Anaemodoron (5 drops 3 times daily before meals with a little water). This remedy stimulates the appetite and helps blood formation. At the same time the mother needs to ensure that the child's diet is regulated: the prime rule is to first let the child go hungry and cleanse the intestines with camomile enemas. To begin with just give fruit juices of all kinds in small quantities, but only as much as the child wishes to drink.

Many mothers are anxious about letting their child go hungry for a few days, as the child may already be 'so thin'. They forget that they have achieved nothing with the dietary approach used so far. In addition the child is unfamiliar with the feeling of 'being hungry', for the parents have probably slipped high-protein morsels into the small amounts the child does eat, or given sweet things or fruit between meals, making it difficult for stomach and liver to recuperate.

But a young child has never yet starved when there was food available; and nor has he remained healthy and in good appetite when forced or induced to eat. All compulsion must be dropped, and parents must be quite relaxed about the issue so that the child loses his disinclination to eat as every mealtime approaches. A child with a poor appetite should be given very little milk, to begin with no more than a quarter of a litre per day. If thirsty, only fruit juice is allowed, never milk.

Every little bit of bread eaten with a good appetite is worth more than a whole meal choked down reluctantly. If, after the first few days of a fruit juice diet a certain desire to eat returns, one can offer rye crackers with just a little butter and cream cheese, or Bircher muesli. If the child asks for milk, give him sour milk, fresh buttermilk or bioyoghurt. The next step is a raw carrot or also steamed vegetables without roux, with just a little fresh butter to begin with.

One gives these foods to the child in very small quantities, and only offers him food three times a day. The child should want food himself and very gradually become accustomed to regular meals and larger quantities. He should never be given sweets instead of food, nor eat anything between meals—not even fruit.

If children do not want to eat breakfast in the mornings, give them a teaspoon of sloe (blackthorn) juice (Weleda or Wala) on an empty stomach, thus stimulating their appetite.

If these home remedies do not work, consult a doctor. There are other homoeopathic and anthroposophical medicines and treatments available which can help.

Jaw deformation (and prevention)

When the teeth start to appear, it is frequently found that bottom and top teeth do not meet properly. If the child sucks his thumb, this condition is made worse. Usually the position adopted by the hand is such that the upper jaw is pushed forwards and the lower backwards. If incisors have already appeared, the upper ones are pushed outwards while the lower ones cannot grow upwards properly. The bottom lip then usually inserts itself between the upper and lower front teeth thus making the situation even worse, so that the child can only bring his lips together with an effort. Air breathed in through the nose is cleaned, warmed, humidified and to a great extent made germ-free. None of this happens when the child breathes through his mouth. In addition, he will tend to swallow air and there will be disturbances and congestion in the blood and lymph circulations of the throat. Faulty positioning and functioning of the mouth and all its parts, combined with faulty breathing, leads to functional, digestive and metabolic disturbances.

Special dummies (NUK-Sauger dummies from Germany) can help prevent these deformations.

But once the jaw is deformed, many years of patient treatment are needed before the situation can be corrected. The best time to start correction is at the change of teeth.

Faulty posture and spinal curvature

Spinal curvature or faulty posture with the resulting damage this can do is often the result of early forced sitting and standing. A child with this problem has a hollow chest, the

spine curves backwards at the top and correspondingly forwards in the small of the back, tilting the pelvis forward and
pushing the abdomen forward. The head is bent forwards and
the shoulders are rounded. The legs are knock-kneed and the
feet flat. The child will need orthopaedic help, and very good
results are also achieved with eurythmy therapy.

Anaemia

Anaemia usually arises from iron deficiency in the blood and
can occur in the first few weeks of life. Those particularly
susceptible are the children of anaemic mothers, premature
babies, babies who are born well after the expected date, and
also twins. The signs are pallor, apathy, tiredness and lack of
appetite. The child is also susceptible to any infections in the
neighbourhood and usually has poor posture.

He will require medical treatment and also dietary help, as
well as a great deal of sun and fresh air.

Nettlerash

Nettlerash and similar allergic reactions will continue to
increase the more we add chemical substances to our food,
our clothes, our washing and cleaning materials, and the
more vaccinations of all kinds are given.

In some cases this can also be an allergy to certain foods,
e.g. strawberries, fish, seafood, or even milk when it touches
the skin, causing eruptions to appear within seconds.

There are a number of preparations the doctor can prescribe for nettlerash. In addition to these, make sure that the
child's bowel and bladder are emptied, and give fresh fruit

and vegetable juice without sugar, as little protein as possible, no white sugar or chocolate or cocoa, very little salt. The itchy parts can be treated with vinegar water ($\frac{2}{3}$ water and $\frac{1}{3}$ wine or cider vinegar), or powder. If the itching persists, give pure cod liver oil ($\frac{1}{2}$ to 1 dessertspoon twice daily). Compresses or baths with Weleda Lavender Bath Lotion (Weleda), or Aesculus Essence (Wala) also help sooth itching.

Eczema

There are many reasons for eczema, which can take numerous forms, for instance red patches of various kinds, lumps, small blisters, scales or scabs. In most cases the cause is an allergy.

It is for the doctor to determine the cause, and the mother should not treat the rash herself with creams or ointments, particularly those containing coal tar or cortisone. Often the liver or spleen are not in order in an eczema sufferer. But disturbances in other organs can also cause skin trouble. Treatment with medicines should always be accompanied by external treatment. Often dietary change will be required. White sugar can cause itching. For some eczemas, milk will have to be avoided (see page 94).

In very persistent cases, the ability of the metabolism to react can be stimulated by a course of 10 to 12 fever-producing baths. This is, for instance, the case with psoriasis.

As a general rule it can be said that weeping rashes should be treated with damp compresses or baths, for instance with Aesculus Essence, and definitely not with greasy ointments. When the irritation has improved, oil or ointments may be useful.

Enlarged tonsils and adenoids

If acute tonsillitis (see pages 148–9), which can occur as early as the first year, is not carefully treated medically until the tonsil swelling has completely subsided, this can be the start of an affliction with enlarged tonsils and/or adenoids which can plague the whole of childhood. The general health of the child can suffer considerably under this strain. It is not sufficiently realized that swollen tonsils and adenoids also block all the passages of the nose, preventing these from being used properly in breathing.

There are a number of natural remedies that can help in treating both acute and chronic tonsillitis. But even with these there are a certain number of failures which have to be treated surgically.

Children who have a tendency towards these inflammations should be taken for their holidays to the mountains or to the seaside. Delicate children will need the warmer resorts, while any coast will suit stronger children.

12

Nursing

It is hoped that the following descriptions of a number of nursing procedures will help the mother to assist the doctor. She should work with him and not on her own without consultation.

Many of these practical nursing traditions are fast disappearing and perhaps these descriptions will help save them from being forgotten forever.

They help the parents to work preventively against illnesses, to alleviate the sick child's distressing symptoms, and to create and maintain a healthy basis for life.

The unrestrained taking of tablets and pills should be seen for what it is, so that people may return to placing their confidence in the healing forces of nature and to an understanding of natural methods of healing.

The mother's love

A baby's healthy development depends to a far higher degree than most mothers realize on the daily intimate contact between mother and child. Far from love being 'just' a vague feeling, the way a child thrives proves that though love may not be visible its effects are recognizable and perceptible.

Babies in hospital are prone to infection just because, despite even the greatest devotion on the part of the nurses, the mother's love is lacking.

Though the physical link with the mother is severed at birth, this is only the very first necessary step on the way to independent existence. The baby still needs the mother's physical proximity as she picks her up in her arms and places her beside her in bed. This encloses the baby ever and again in motherly warmth so that she is totally surrounded by the mood the mother creates. Only the mother completely and utterly understands her child's needs which are at first almost wholly physical but soon become psychological as well.

Children who are separated from their mother during the first year, for whatever reason, suffer damage without any doubt, and only the most devoted care by other people can hope to compensate for this to some degree. Every unnecessary absence of the mother should therefore be avoided. Some forms of schizophrenia can now be in some part attributed to disruption of the links between mother and child in early infancy.

If possible it is also advisable not to move house until the child is weaned and has become somewhat more independent. Every place has its own atmosphere. Frequent or major change at an early age is not beneficial for the young child's calm, even development.

Behaviour and facial expressions of the sick child

When a child falls sick suddenly, it is useful for the doctor if the mother can describe the child's behaviour and expression when she telephones him or as soon as he arrives.

The way the child shows she is in pain is particularly revealing. It is difficult to glean anything from the baby's face, since if she is screaming it will be bright red, while her mouth will be wide open and her eyes screwed shut. She is likely to howl with abandon regardless of whether the pain is in her tummy, head, ears or even just the mucous membranes in her mouth as a result of teething. If the pain is due to teething, she will be trying to stuff her little fist into her mouth. Abdominal pain (colic) will make her draw up her legs suddenly and then push away again with her feet, and her tummy will be as hard as a board. Thus her limbs show us where the pain is situated. Earache will make her throw her head to and fro while she clumsily tries to stroke the painful ear. If she is crying because of pneumonia, which can be very painful owing to the accompanying pleurisy, her mouth will hardly be open but her eyes will be wide open and shiny with fever. Her eyebrows will be drawn up in a frown and her mouth turned down at the corners. The pain in the pleura will force her to dampen the actual screaming. Characteristic breathing is the most important sign of pneumonia, since the doctor can often not hear anything through his stethoscope while the illness is still confined to the inner recesses of the lungs. From time to time, or constantly, the child breathes out in an audible sigh while the nostrils open wide. Peritonitis causes quick, shallow breathing interspersed with an occasional deep sighing exhalation. A child with meningitis wears a determined, thoughtful, rather fixed and serious expression. Her eyes will be sensitive to light, which in turn leads to a vertical frown on the brow. Her glance is absent and mouth firmly shut except when she occasionally emits a piercing scream. The limbs are usually still. A small child with pyelonephritis usually makes small agitated movements with her trunk, hollowing or even arching her back, and also makes strange twisting movements with her hands, whose palms are burning hot.

Mention has already been made of the characteristic sleep position of the healthy child, with her arms raised one on either side of her head, and of the sick child whose arms lie at her sides. Remember also that the delicate perfume of small babies fades at the onset of an illness.

Observation of the child's behaviour continues to be most important for the doctor well beyond infancy, since most two- or three-year-olds are still unable to give useful information as to 'where it hurts'. Some children who have had uncomfortable experiences with the doctor will also try to dissemble in order to avoid examination or another bout of treatment.

The doctor's diagnosis is also helped by observing the type of cough (dry, cramped, moist, sighing, hollow or whooping) or the type and consistency of vomiting (spluttering, pouring, with slime or the contents of the stomach, or with blood or consisting entirely of blood), as well as urine and faeces. Samples of excretions from bladder, bowel, vagina, nose or ears should be preserved for the doctor.

Taking the temperature

Ascertaining the exact temperature is very important and with small children taking the temperature in the rectum is the most reliable method, though if the child struggles this is virtually impossible. However, if she has been used to this method from infancy she will not be afraid and there is absolutely no need for the method to be painful. Hold the well greased thermometer lightly between thumb and forefinger and insert into the rectum. It is best for a small baby to lie on her back while you hold her feet up with your free hand. Older children can lie on their side or tummy.

Older children can have their temperature taken in the mouth (under the tongue). Taking the temperature under the arm is not suitable with children as they cannot grip the thermometer tightly enough. Sometimes the temperature can be taken in the groin. The mercury should be well shaken down and the thermometer is kept in place for at least five minutes.

If appendicitis is suspected, take the temperature under the arm first, making sure that the child grips the thermometer tightly. Then take the temperature again in the rectum. The normal difference between external and internal temperature is 0.35°F (0.5°C). If the internal temperature is more than 0.35°F above the external measurement, an abdominal inflammation can be suspected. The doctor should be called, even at night, and told of the difference between the measurements.

There is no point taking the temperature within two hours after a meal, as digestion usually causes the temperature to rise. The best times are in the morning when the child wakes and in the afternoon between 3.30 and 4.30. (See also *The healing power of fever*, pages 120–1.)

Diet during acute illness

The main rule as regards diet in any acute illness, whether feverish or not, is to give little food. Feed the child only if she wants something and do not give so-called 'nourishing food', i.e. meat, broth or eggs. It is better to go hungry, because the digestive juices in mouth, stomach and intestines are greatly reduced or even absent in acute illness. Food is therefore not properly digested and only causes discomfort. All the child's forces are needed to combat the illness and it is not serious if some weight is lost. Most of this weight is fluid, which is easily lost when the child is ill or has a temperature but is just as easily restored afterwards, especially if the child's appetite has not been spoiled for months ahead by having been forced to eat.

It is best to offer small amounts of fresh fruit juices and fresh fruit, e.g. oranges, apples, berries or whatever is in season. Take care to peel sprayed fruits!

If the stomach is not affected by the illness and there is no vomiting or diarrhoea, the child can have warm milk. It is best to remove the cream and dilute the milk with herb tea or mineral water since this makes it more digestible. Grain coffee with a little honey can also be recommended. If the doctor does not specify, give very weak ordinary tea or preferably camomile, peppermint, rose hip or yarrow tea. Give no or very little sugar. (So-called glucose is usually made by a cheap chemical method from maize and has no special value.) Honey in small amounts is best. This should be added to the beverage when it is cool enough to drink, since temperatures over 104°F (40°C) spoil its health-giving properties.

Milk encourages mucous and should therefore only be given diluted to children with throat infections or bronchial catarrh. Small babies, however, must not go without milk for more than three days during the first nine months unless the doctor gives instructions to this effect. Older children with a high temperature often have an aversion to fresh milk but might take it diluted or else might like sour milk, buttermilk, yogurt, kefir or similar products. If not, give them fruit juice or plain mineral water.

A child with a temperature needs more liquids. Let her have as much as she wants, but make her sip it slowly. Stewed apple and other cooked fruit may also be given if the illness has not affected the stomach. Sugar should be added in small amounts only, since otherwise there is a danger of diarrhoea or a vitamin deficiency. Fresh fruit is usually preferred and better.

For the main meals try offering a cup of oat or semolina gruel, especially if you can obtain Demeter or other good brands. Rusks, biscuits and bread should also be made from good flour. White wheat or rye flour has no nutritional value. This provides no vitamins for the sick person, indeed it even robs her of her small supply of vitamin B when it has to be digested. So a small amount of good bread with a little butter or good vegetable margarine (no additives!) is better than twice the amount of white bread or biscuits.

The medicine chest

Every household needs a well-stocked medicine chest containing both remedies for illness and first aid equipment for accidents. It should be placed out of the reach of children and securely locked. A note of the doctor's and chemist's telephone number pinned on the inside of the door is useful. It should contain a book of instructions on first aid for injuries and poisoning. (For the treatment of wounds, see page 189.)

Well-sealed remedies, both liquids and also powders and tablets, can be kept for years. The following list may be used as a guide:

Thermometer

Scissors

Tweezers (large and small)

Feeding cup

Hot water bottle

Safety pin (several sizes)

Leather finger stall

Compresses

Sling

Medicine spoon

Pipette

Kidney bowl

Balloon enema

Enema for children and adults

Cotton wool (large pack)

Bandages

Lint

Gauzes of various sizes

Melolin dressings (non-stick)

W.C.S. Powder (Weleda)

Combudoron (liquid and ointment) (Weleda) for burns

Arnica ointment 10% (Weleda) for sprains

Arnica essence 20% for damp compresses for bruises

Mercurialis ointment 10% for bad bruises and as a drawing
    ointment (also useful as a nose cream for children!)

Weleda Balsamicum ointment

Calendula essence 20% for damp compresses on open
    wounds and for rinsing the mouth for bleeding gums

Valerian drops for overexcitement and sleeplessness.
    Adults 20 drops on a lump of sugar. Babies 4 drops in
    sugar water

Melissa comp. (Weleda) drops to be taken for stomach upsets and spells of faintness, and used externally for headaches, earaches, etc.

Compresses and water treatments

The general rule is that baths or other applications of cold water should only be made to parts of the body that are sufficiently warm. Also, cold water is only suitable if its use engenders a comforting glow. If the patient does not warm up sufficiently, her circulation can be stimulated by massaging with a brush. If the circulation in the skin improves, the massage can be followed by a quick rub down with cold water.

THE UTENSILS

Containers: A bath or large basin

Wraps and towels: For chest, throat and calf compresses three different cloths are needed. The size will depend on the child's age.

1. The inner cloth is placed wet next to the skin. Rough linen or wild silk are the most suitable materials. The width for throat compresses should be the length of the throat (it must reach up to the ears), and for chest compresses it should reach from under the arms down to the buttocks. Calf compresses must cover the whole calf.

2. The next cloth should also be linen (not cotton). It should be larger above and below than the inner and the outer cloth so that on the one hand the wet inner cloth never

protrudes and on the other the woollen outer cloth never touches the skin. Both are uncomfortable for the sick person.

3. The outer cloth is of thick wool or flannel. It should be an inch or two wider than the inner cloth so that no cold air reaches the inner compresses. On the other hand it should be smaller than the middle cloth so that it does not touch the patient's skin.

The cloths should be long enough to go about $1\frac{1}{2}$ times round throat, chest or calf respectively. They may be prepared when the child is well and kept in readiness for when they may be needed. Waterproof material is never necessary.

WASHINGS

This is best done when the child is nice and warm on waking in the morning or when she is really warm in bed in the evening. Fold a coarse hand towel several times and wring out lightly after dipping in cold water. Rub vigorously from the back of the right hand up the outside of the arm to the shoulder and then down again along the inside of the arm to the palm. Do the same with the left arm. If necessary wet the towel again. Wash neck, chest and back with a few strokes. Then starting on top of the right foot wash up the outside of the leg to the buttock and back down the inside to the sole of the foot. Do the same with the other leg and wash vigorously between the legs. The tummy is washed last. The whole operation should take only a few seconds. Put on the night clothes without drying and cover up snugly in bed. If the child does not glow with a cosy warmth at the latest after 10–

20 minutes, the washing was done too slowly or the room was not warm enough.

Instead of washing the child all over in one sitting, either her upper or lower half can be washed. Usually you would start with her arms and upper part and go on to washing the whole child after a few days.

COMPRESSES

General remarks: Compresses can be applied to throat, arms, chest, loins, legs, calves and feet. The patient must lie in bed during the application.

Damp, hot compresses release cramp and thus relieve pain. The bed and cloths must be well warmed before the compress is applied.

Cold-water compresses (50°–68°F (10–20°C) are used on the one hand to reduce body temperature (the heat is absorbed in the cloths), and on the other to make the patient perspire. To reduce body temperature the inner cloth should be left rather wet. To induce sweating it should be well wrung out, which will cause warmth to build up until the patient breaks into perspiration. When this happens, the compress (which should have no air pockets) is removed. If the compress is too wet or if the water was lukewarm instead of cold, it can happen that the child fails to heat it up. In this case it must be removed immediately and the child rubbed with a Turkish towel to warm her. She may need a hot drink of lime-blossom tea as well.

Cold calf compresses are left for 20 minutes and then repeated three to five times at 20-minute intervals. This is usually sufficient to draw the fever down from the head. The patient's discomfort is thus relieved and her face is no longer so hot and red. The compresses should stop when the temperature has been reduced to about 101.3°F (38.5°C), since this will be sufficient to relieve the headache due to pressure of blood in the head.

Cold throat compresses must reach up to the ears and must not be too loose or they will not get warm. As with calf compresses, they can be repeated several times a day.

Hot mustard compresses applied properly and soon enough can relieve pneumonia (and its early stages) dramatically. Stir a heaped dessertspoon of freshly ground mustard (it should have a piercing smell) into a pint of almost boiling water. Dip the inner cloth in this and let it steep. Remove with a wooden spoon and as soon as you can bear to touch it, apply it to the child's chest or to the side affected. Quickly wrap the other cloths round it. After no more than ten minutes, look to see if the skin is bright red. If it is, remove the compress immediately and wash the reddened skin carefully with lukewarm water. Similarly, remove immediately if the child cries in pain. Left too long, the compress can burn the skin. Finally powder the skin (for instance with Weleda WCS powder).

COLD AND HOT COMPRESSES

Cold compresses should be as cold as possible, never lukewarm. They must never be applied to cold skin. Hot compresses should be as hot as bearable.

Cold compresses made with several layers of well-wrung cloths reduce bleeding and swelling and relieve pain where there are injuries, bruises and contusions. These compresses are not covered with woollen outer cloths. They are renewed as soon as they start to warm up, and repeated as long as they bring relief.

Cooling compresses (possibly with a little wine vinegar) can be placed on the heart to calm the patient. A compress on the back of the neck stems a nose bleed and also calms the heart of a nervous person.

Wounds, for instance children's cuts and grazes, should never be washed, even if they are covered in dirt. Gently pour some water over the place to rinse away the movable pieces of grit and then cover with dry linen or gauze. This is then dampened repeatedly but not removed. The water used for this can contain Calendula Essence 20% (Weleda or Wala), or Arnica Essence. A weak salt solution of $\frac{1}{4}$ oz (9g) salt to 2 pints (1 litre) water will also do if necessary. The wound needs the greatest possible quiet to enable it to repel the dirt and bacteria.

For burns, Combudoron Lotion (Weleda) is added to the water in accordance with the instructions on the bottle.

Hot compresses are used to relieve painful cramps, for instance gall, stomach and kidney colics. It is a mistake to treat these conditions, which come and go in waves, with an electric blanket or dry hot water bottles. These compresses are also good for menstrual pains in girls and for softening boils, carbuncles and abscesses. They can also be used for bronchitis, pleurisy and inflammation of the joints. Whooping cough, croup and asthma can often be relieved as well.

If hayflowers (flores graminis) are obtainable, make a bag of the required size out of strong material and fill this with the flowers to make a thickness of about 2 inches (5cm). Place the filled bag in a bowl and pour on enough boiling water to saturate the flowers without making the bag dripping wet. (Wring the bag gently if you put on too much.) If it is well covered up, the bag will hold its warmth for at least an hour. It is very effective and soothing especially for inflamed joints and also for abdominal colics (though for the latter it should not be too heavy).

BATHS

As a rule, late morning and later afternoon are the most suitable times for baths, while the most unsuitable is just before or just after a main meal. Three baths a week is the normal requirement, unless otherwise prescribed.

Warm baths: Temperature between 95 and 98.6°F (35–37°C). Bath mixtures made from pine needles, camomile, sloes, rosemary, valerian, kalmus, lavender, sulphur, are used to strengthen or calm the patient or for the treatment of the skin. For duration, see under hot baths.

Hot baths: Temperature between 100.4 and 104°F (38–40°C). Baths whose temperature is gradually raised are very effective in the early stages of colds, bronchitis and flu.

The patient should stay in the warm or hot bath for 10 to 15 minutes. After this, wash or rinse her down with cool water to close the pores opened by the warmth. The bath is followed by three hours in bed.

Schlenz Baths: This method was developed by Frau Maria Schlenz in Innsbruck. It is also described as a warming bath. It can be applied at the beginning of or during acute feverish illnesses such as tonsillitis, flu, incipient pneumonia, bronchitis, pyelonephritis, etc. Professor Lampert of Höxter treated serious infectious diseases such as spotted typhoid, dysentery and typhoid by this method and I myself have treated soldiers seriously ill with kidney disease in the field hospital in Prague during the war, even when they had high blood pressure. Acute lumbago can be healed in the shortest time and the method is indispensable for the improvement of some chronic complaints and also for the paralysis after polio.

Method: It is important to be very exact. The patient's bowel is emptied with the help of an enema, after which her temperature is taken. The water temperature at the beginning is made to correspond with this. Stick the end of the thermometer into a piece of cork and let it hang in the water. (Take care: at a temperature of over 107.6°F (42°C) it will burst!)

A decoction of hayflowers (flores graminis) is added to the bath water. For an adult, brew 10–14 oz (300–400g) hayflowers in hot water in a bag and let it draw (use less for a child). Pour the decoction into the bath, keeping the bag as a head rest. The patient lies stretched out in the bath with her head on the bag. Her neck must be covered by the water which reaches almost to her mouth.

During the first 15 minutes gradually raise the temperature of the water (by using a boiling kettle) to 101.3°F (38.5°C). This serves to open the pores and prepare the patient for the effects of the bath. After this the patient should be warned that she will go through a few minutes of discomfort. Her pulse will race and she will feel all the parts that have been affected by the illness. This is the sign that the organism is beginning to react. It may help to scrub the patient's skin with a brush or let her sit up for a moment. This slightly alarming state soon passes and the patient begins to feel uncomfortable in the bath. The temperature can now gradually be increased to 102°F (39°C). Do not make it any hotter for the patient's first such bath, but maintain this temperature for the rest of the hour which the bath should take. Children often react more quickly and the bath can be ended when they have had beads of sweat on their forehead for some time. But for the full effect the bath should last an hour. Then it is gradually brought to an end. The patient sits up and is then helped to stand up. She is wrapped in a large towel and put straight into bed without drying, where she should sweat for another hour well covered up.

After an hour wash the patient with lukewarm water to which you can add a little vinegar. Put on dry clothes and put her straight back to bed. Now is the time for a glass of orange juice or other fresh fruit juice. The perspiration will have brought about a considerable loss of vitamin C which must quickly be replaced. Other suitable drinks are rose hip tea, orange or lemon tea sweetened with honey, Sandthorn Elixir or other Weleda or Wala elixirs.

The Schlenz Bath can also be given as a footbath, for instance for flu, sinusitis, etc. The warmly wrapped patient sits with her feet in a deep bowl or bucket. The hayflower decoction is added and should lead to strong perspiration all over the body, lasting for an hour.

For the second or third bath the water temperature can be increased to 103.1°F (39.5°C) or more, as long as the patient is still comfortable. After a night's sleep she will feel born anew. This bath method has the strongest effect of all water applications. It is particularly suitable when a rapid recovery is required or when an illness drags on for a long time because the patient's forces of resistance are insufficient.

Alternating baths: For children, alternating baths should only be given as foot or arm baths. The feet or arms are warmed first in warm water at 102.2°F (39°C) for three to five minutes and then immersed in cold water at 46–50°F (8–10°C) for ten seconds. This is repeated three to five times, but from the second time onwards only two minutes are necessary for the warm, followed again by ten seconds immersion in the cold water. The treatment ends with a quick rinse in cold water to close the pores, and the child is then put straight to bed wrapped in a towel (without drying) where she will soon begin to glow with warmth. (Cold water should never be applied to skin that is already cold.)

These baths are particularly suitable for children suffering from cold feet or hands. The series of hot and cold immersions can be done with the feet on one day and with the arms on the next and so on. Such baths are particularly important for youngsters during puberty and in the case of bladder or other abdominal weakness, and also for headache and sleeplessness. Parents should not take it lightly if their children always have cold feet, since this can be the root of a number of serious weaknesses and illnesses.

Regarding daily bathing, see pages 74–5.

POULTICES
Poultices resemble compresses but do not involve the use of water.

Beeswax poultice: This is used for bronchitis and bad coughs which disturb sleep at night. The beeswax (about 50g for babies and small children) is melted in hot water, on which it floats. A piece of linen is dipped in the melted wax and then quickly placed on chest or back (both if possible) and covered in warm wrappings to keep it hot for as long as possible. The poultice can be left on overnight and is very comforting, relieving the coughing.

Onion poultice: Sudden pain of the middle ear in babies and small children is relieved within a few minutes by this poultice. Chop a medium-sized onion and put in a muslin bag. Place this on the ear, allowing it to overlap on all sides. Cover with a good layer of cotton wool and keep in position with a balaclava helmet. Relief is almost immediate. If it is not, the doctor must be called straight away.

Fenugreek poultice: This works as a drawing paste. The seeds of this plant are used to draw the pus from inflammations (boils, abscesses, etc.). Boil one or two dessertspoons in water to form a thick paste. A layer ($\frac{3}{4}$ inch thick) is placed while as hot as possible on the centre of the boil and left covered with cotton wool till it cools. The treatment is repeated till the pus is discharged, which happens relatively quickly and painlessly, with very little damage to the skin. Lancing can often be avoided in this way.

Appendix One

Bottles and Teats

The glass or plastic baby's bottle is graded showing amounts up to 200g. Larger amounts would be unsuitable and might tempt the mother to give the baby more than 200g at one feed.

The bottle has a rubber cap. Immediately after a meal both are rinsed in cold water and the bottle is left standing full of water. Once a day bottles and caps are washed with a bottle brush in hot water with soda, after which they are rinsed in hot water and left to drip dry. If washing-up liquid is used they must be very thoroughly rinsed with hot water so there is no risk of contaminating the next meal with detergent.

The teat should as closely as possible resemble the nipple. Usually it is already pierced, but if not this can be done with a glowing darning needle. The hole or holes should be just large enough to allow the food to drip through. The drink must not run too easily into the baby's mouth. As with the breast, the baby should have to make a certain effort to obtain the milk.

After every meal the teat is washed thoroughly in cold water to which a little salt may be added. It is then kept in a clean jar with a lid. Both jar and teats must be boiled daily for three minutes. Never touch the end of the teat with the fingers. The smallest remnants of food left in bottle or teat can become the breeding ground for germs which can even endanger life.

Appendix Two

Utensils for Bottle Feeding

1 milk saucepan large enough to boil one pint of milk
1 enamel saucepan (to hold about 2 pints) for cooking Holle baby food
2–5 graded baby bottles with rubber caps
1 hair sieve for sieving the baby food
1–2 rubber teats with holes
1 bottle brush
1 small saucepan for boiling the teats and the jar in which they are kept
1 glass jar with lid for storing teats
Soda crystals for washing

It is also useful to have:

a stand for drip-drying the bottles
a measuring jug (glass) graded up to 250 or even 500g

All these utensils should be used exclusively for the baby's food.

Appendix Three

Preparing Holle Baby Food

The gruel
The amount of food to be used is shown on the packet. Mix the food (Holle Oat Flakes, Holle No. 1 or Holle No. 2) with the amount of water shown and boil for about two minutes, stirring constantly. The gruel is ready when it emits a delicious smell of fresh bread. The cooking time can be increased for babies who do not digest too easily. If the baby is not breastfed, it is best to start with oat gruel for the first month and change to Holle No. 1 during the second month. This gruel is then used to make the mixtures below.

Half milk, half gruel mixture
Example: Add 100g of the gruel together with two teaspoons of ordinary sugar to 100g of separately boiled milk. The amount for the whole day can be prepared in the morning. After mixing thoroughly it is put into the feeding bottles which are kept in the fridge with their caps on. A bottle is then heated in a water bath when the meal is due.

Two thirds milk, one third gruel mixture
For example 100g is added to 50g gruel. Sweetening and storing of the day's supply as above.

Feeding
Shake the bottle well and then heat up in a water bath. The correct temperature is ascertained by touching your eyelid

with the bottle or letting a drop fall on the back of your hand. On no account try sucking the teat. If the baby drinks slowly, the bottle will have to be reheated during the meal, possibly more than once.

Appendix Four

How to Make Curd Cheese

Warm the milk to blood heat and add a spoonful of either sour milk or live yogurt. The bacteria are different, but both result in a souring and thickening of the milk. Allow to stand in a warm place till the milk has thickened. Pour into a muslin or cheese bag and suspend over a bowl for about twelve hours while the whey drains away. The resulting crumbly curds can be used as they are or made smooth by adding fresh cream or milk and whisking gently with a hand whisk.

This is added to the baby's main meal and is the best way of providing his protein needs. For older children and adults it is delicious mixed with finely chopped herbs and eaten on bread or with vegetables. Mixed with chopped fruit or fruit juice it makes a popular dessert.

Appendix Five

How to Make Almond Milk

(The Granovita company supplies almond pulp, which is rather laborious to make oneself—www.granovita.de)

For milk-free bottle feeding with almond pulp and lactose:

	Daily amount	
	300 ml (shared between 2–6 bottles)	600 ml (shared between 3–6 bottles)
Water (see Appendix Six) 6–7% almond pulp 6% lactose★	300 ml 18–21g 18g	600 ml 36–42g 36g

Method: Mix the above in boiled water.

For 1/3 milk with almond paste and lactose:

	Daily amount		
	600 ml (shared between 4–6 bottles)	750 ml (shared between 4–5 bottles)	900 ml (shared between 4–5 bottles)
1 part cow's milk 2 parts water (see next appendix) 4% almond pulp 6% lactose★	200 ml 400 ml 24g 36g	250 ml 500 ml 30g 45g	300 ml 600 ml 36g 54g

★ Corresponds to the sugar content of mother's milk and cannot be replaced by any other sugar.

Method: Boil milk and water together briefly (to at least 80°C). Stir the almond pulp with a little warm water and add to the milk together with the lactose, without allowing it to boil. Sieve and share between bottles. After cooling in cold water, bottles for the day must be stored in the fridge. The bottles should not contain more feed than the child should receive, i.e. no more than 1/7 to 1/6 of the body weight.

Appendix Six

Water Quality

Normal tap-water generally contains too much nitrate and chlorine and should therefore not be used for preparing baby food. Water from old lead pipes can also contain considerable quantities of lead.

Mineral water may not be suitable either, if it has too high a salt and mineral content.

Volvic water from the Auvergne region of France has a low mineral content and can therefore be recommended for baby food.

It is also preferable to use water from glass rather than plastic bottles, as bacteria often proliferate in plastic bottles, and the plastic, also, is said to give off oestrogen hormones.

Spring water is also doubtless good, although, since it is not subject to checks and controls, it might not be clean.

Appendix Seven

Reducing the Risk of Cot Death

Very occasionally babies die suddenly for no obvious reason, from what is called 'cot death' or 'sudden infant death syndrome' (SIDS). Although the causes are still unclear, placing a baby to sleep on his or her back reduces the risk, as does ensuring a cigarette smoke-free environment. Another possible contributory factor is overheating.

Below is a comprehensive list of all steps you can take to diminish the risk of cot death.

Sleeping place and position:

- Always put your baby to sleep on his or her back, unless a doctor has advised otherwise for specific reasons.
- Keep your baby's cot in your bedroom for the first six months or so
- Don't use plastic sheets or have ribbons or bits of string (e.g. mobiles) near the cot where your baby can get caught in them.
- Make sure there is no gap between the cot mattress and the side of the cot through which your baby can slip down.
- Make sure the mattress is firm, flat and clean. The outside of the mattress should be waterproof, but not have any loose plastic covering that could come off and choke your baby. Fire-retardant materials found in some cot mattresses

are probably best avoided, though no direct link with cot death has been proved.

- Use sheets and lightweight blankets but not duvets, quilts, bedding rolls or pillows etc.
- Don't leave your baby to sleep propped up on a cushion on a sofa, or in an armchair.

Overheating:

- Don't let your baby get too hot and don't overheat the room. If the room is warm enough for you to be comfortable in light clothing, this is the right temperature for your baby too (16–20°C).
- Keep your baby's head uncovered in bed. A baby needs to lose heat from his or her head and face. By placing your baby in the 'feet to foot' position (with his/her feet right at the end of the cot), you prevent the baby wriggling under the covers.
- Remove hats and extra clothing whenever you come indoors or enter a warm place (e.g. a train or car).
- If you take your baby into your bed to sleep, make sure he/she is not too hot under your duvet.
- Never give the baby a hot water bottle or an electric blanket.
- If your baby is feverish, don't give him or her extra bedding.

Smoking:

- Stop smoking in pregnancy. This also applies to fathers! (Babies and young children exposed to cigarette smoke are also more susceptible to coughs, asthma and chest/ear infections.)

- No one should smoke in the same room as your baby.
- If you are a smoker it is possible that sharing your bed with a baby may increase the risk of cot death.

In general, always ask for a doctor's advice quickly if your baby seems at all unwell. Cot death is rare—take the precautions listed above but don't let fear of it spoil the first precious months with your baby.

Further Reading

Health:

An Introduction to Anthroposophical Medicine, Victor Bott (Sophia Books)

Medicine, An Introductory Reader, Rudolf Steiner (Sophia Books)

A Guide to Child Health, Michaela Glockler and Wolfgang Goebel (Floris Books)

Sound Sleep, Sarah Woodhouse (Hawthorn Press)

Education:

An Introduction to Steiner Education, Francis Edmunds (Sophia Books)

Education, An Introductory Reader, Rudolf Steiner (Sophia Books)

The Education of the Child, Rudolf Steiner (SteinerBooks)

The Developing Child, Sense and Nonsense in Education, Willi Aeppli (SteinerBooks)

The Incarnating Child, Joan Salter (Hawthorn Press)